Psychedelics
Dreams
& Rituals

Published by Lisa Hagan Books 2023

www.lisahaganbooks.com

Cover and interior layout by Simon Hartshorne

Psychedelics
Dreams
& Rituals

A Guidebook for Explorers, Therapists, and Facilitators

GAY LYNN GRIGAS, LMHC

Endorsements

"Excellent guidebook written by a MAPS-trained and licensed therapist working in the field."
—**Rick Doblin, Ph.D.**, Founder and President of MAPS

"Here is a well-researched and well-grounded guidebook and workbook for anyone motivated to seriously cultivate personal development and spiritual awakening. Enjoy!"
—**William A. (Bill) Richards,Ph.D.**, *Sacred Knowledge: Psychedelics and Religious Experiences*

"As a licensed and trained psychedelic therapist, Gay Lynn shares her expertise on how to use psychedelics, dreams, and rituals for inner healing. Through her workshops, groups, and individual sessions she guides people to their own healing of trauma and how to deal effectively with their anxiety and depression. Gay Lynn is truly a gifted therapist."
—**Eric Milbrandt, MD,** Oasis Wellness & Recovery

"Having worked for several years in the fields of neurosciences, mental health, and clinical research, I decided to take the next step to psychedelic therapies when I had the privilege to meet Gay Lynn during our MAPS therapist training. Gay Lynn is an exceptional human being and a truly gifted psychedelic therapist. As I got to know her and worked together, I witnessed her spiritual wisdom, therapeutic knowledge, and skills which are extremely valuable for work with expanded states of consciousness. In *Psychedelics, Dreams, and Rituals: A Guidebook for Explorers, Therapists, and Facilitators* she shares her best practices providing invaluable guidance to help people take their inner healing journey. I wholeheartedly recommend this book to beginner explorers as well as therapists and facilitators doing psychedelic work with individuals and groups."
—**Fabiana da Silva Alves, Ph.D.,** Psychedelic Therapist, The Netherlands

"In our rush for efficiency and explosive growth, our modern world has lost its sacredness. Today's epidemic of loneliness and disconnection is the unfortunate fruit of this headlong rush into the future, without regard for the past. In this time of crisis and chaos, psychedelic medicine has made a timely resurgence. However psychedelic medicine is about much more than just the substance and we risk losing the deepest wisdom of these medicines if we try to make psychedelics fit into the model of Western allopathic medicine. What is needed now is the sacredness and deep care that comes with the indigenous traditions of using these medicines to work with non-ordinary states of consciousness in an intentional and respectful way. Gay Lynn has brought together the elements of medicine work, dreams, and rituals in a way that is both honoring the ways

of the past and infused with fresh, modern perspectives. She provides grounded, insightful suggestions and essential reflection questions for working with non-ordinary states in her excellent workbook, written with both clinicians and journeyers in mind. She shares a wealth of ideas that are well-planned from her decades of experience facilitating groups and individual counseling. Gay Lynn shares how to explore non-ordinary states of consciousness to support inner healing experiences utilizing psychedelics, dreams, and rituals. I recommend this creative and engaging book to deepen your exploration and healing endeavors."
— **Linnea Butler, LMFT,** Founder-Bay Area Mental Health

"A book that goes beyond 'set and setting' by a huge leap and describes in detail how to structure working with dreams and 'non-ordinary' states to address trauma and life's many deeper inquiries toward a unified Self. As a student of life, my soul, and my psyche, I cannot recommend this book highly enough to all lifelong searchers looking to refine and add significantly to their quest for rich understanding and new perspectives from within - a most worthy effort aided by a truly connected author/guide who enriches us with a three synthesis of important modalities and states which are deeply helpful and thoughtfully described herein."
—**Pam Olsen, JD, MS**

"For the last nine months I have had the privilege and honor of living and experiencing -- yes, 'live and in person' -- the process you are about to discover in this book. Even saying it was "life-changing" is the understatement of my life. I am a completely different person than I was when I first started this process. When I first started working with Gay Lynn, my life had descended into chaos and despair. I felt like a complete basket case. I had been a police officer in the inner city at the very start of the crack cocaine epidemic. And had the scars -- physical and emotional -- to prove it. I had also just gone through a sudden and unexpected breakup of my marriage. With Ketamine Assisted Psychotherapy and Gay Lynn's methods you are about to discover in this book, that I am relieved of PTSD, chronic pain, anxiety, and depression. All of which had plagued me -- at times it was debilitating -- for more than three decades.

But that is only the tip of the iceberg. The spiritual insights, and consequential spiritual growth, that have happened during this process have been amazing. I am excited that you get to experience Gay Lynn's talent, experience, and expertise in this book. If you only get 1 percent as much from it as I have, it will still be one of the most impactful things you have ever done."
—**Dan Gallapoo,** a former Law Enforcement Officer, participated in clinical work at Oasis Wellness & Recovery, Ocala, FL.

CONTENTS

The ideas in this book should not be interpreted as a substitute for proper medical or psychological treatment. See a physician or trained therapist when you have questions about any aspect of your health or when you need medical or psychological care.

Use this book's information about psychedelics, dreams, and rituals in conjunction with the most effective methods of medicine and psychotherapy while under the direct supervision of a health care provider.

The intent of this book is only to provide information and the author's experience and opinions regarding experiences in a therapeutic and medical clinic with an appropriate set and setting. Before taking any treatments, a medical evaluation is needed to determine if this is a suggested treatment modality based on a professional review of medical and psychological history.

Readers should be aware that currently, in the U.S., most psychedelics are Schedule I controlled substances, which are illegal, and using, buying, or selling them can and will have legal ramifications. Additionally, be aware that psychedelic substances, including ketamine, should not be used for therapy with individuals with ketamine addictions, pregnant women or nursing mothers, people with a history of psychosis or schizophrenia, active hypomania, or poorly controlled high blood pressure.

The author and publisher assume no responsibility for any treatments a reader elects to undergo based on any information or opinions in this book.

Introduction Overview: Healing the Pain of Trauma

This book is your guide to inner healing.

Trauma is a part of so many of our lives today. You may have experienced trauma, but it does not have to define your life. Trauma is a "part" but not a "whole" of our existence. Family trauma may have a generational arch that spans over decades but can be overcome. Trauma is an event that scares us and scars us; however, we can heal.

This book delivers new and accessible pathways for inner healing. This book comes from the perspective that there is an innate healing wisdom within us, an inner healer, a presence, and a power that can and will help us to restore ourselves. The three pathways to enter this healing journey are a combination of psychedelics, dreams, and rituals. These three pathways, used with intention and an experienced therapist or facilitator, can free us to live more fully and freely beyond trauma. This is your detailed guidebook to inner healing. And for a while, I will be your expert guide, and we will take this journey together.

Where Aldous Huxley meets Dr. Carl Jung, where "The Doors of Perception" meets "Memories, Dreams, and Reflections." By entering the non-ordinary state of consciousness using psychedelic medicine, discovering our dream realm, and tapping into the healing power of rituals. The three woven together are what

I call the triune cord. Every single cord of psychedelic medicines, dreams, and rituals is a cord for healing. Woven together, they strengthen and integrate one another for the best potential healing from inner pain and suffering at the deepest levels of our being. Used together, they are like a three-strand cord, which is the strongest and cannot be easily broken.

FOR BEGINNER EXPLORERS TO PROFESSIONALS

This guidebook is for beginners and professionals who understand the power of three healing pathways when we learn how to use them individually and together. This book is written from some of my own stories and my healing journey. Additionally, it chronicles my work as a psychotherapist, working with thousands of healing experiences with hundreds of people suffering from trauma, anxiety, and depression for over thirty years of my career. As the Director of Psychedelic Assisted Therapies now in Ocala, Florida, I work with Ketamine Assisted Psychotherapy. I share some of my therapeutic solutions, the simplest and best practices, and what I believe are the most effective ways to enter our own inner healing experiences.

SEEING THE TRAUMA FROM OUTSIDE THE JAR

I am also a Credentialed Addiction Professional, and paradoxically I am suggesting that using psychedelic substances and entering non-ordinary states will help us to heal trauma. The paradox of entering non-ordinary states to go beyond the threshold of the ego and default mode is the epiphany and the breakthrough needed to begin to know our true selves and view our personal stories from the broadest perspectives. Psychedelic medicine does not so much alter perceptions as it does broaden perceptions. It is like seeing the Earth from outer space. For the first time, we see the whole Earth.

With psychedelic medicine, we get to see our trauma from outside the jar of our life. When we are inside the jar of our pain and suffering from trauma, it is hard, if not impossible, to see outside the jar. When we are in it, trauma, pain, and agony are all we can see and feel. The non-ordinary state of consciousness with psychedelic medicine takes us out of the jar, and we get a chance to look at the jar from the outside and reflect on it from a new perspective. This new perspective is a wider view and can be immensely helpful and healing. This new perspective often creates greater empathy for us and others. By doing so, we become a more real and authentic version of ourselves. We become kinder to ourselves and show up more fully with self-compassion and self-forgiveness. We also discover a new awareness of others from a broader perspective from outside the jar.

WELL-BEING AND MENTAL HEALTH

Mental health is essential at every stage of our lives. It includes our emotional, psychological, and social well-being and impacts how we think, feel, and act. When we have good mental health, we can handle stress better, have better interpersonal relationships, and make healthier choices. Yet today, we are at a crossroads. Despite the advances in therapy, medicine, and healthcare delivery, mental health issues continue to be at epidemic proportions, from addictions to anxiety and depression to eating disorders and Post Traumatic Stress Disorder (PTSD). According to the US Centers for Disease Control and Prevention, mental illnesses are among the most common, as the statistics reveal:

- More than 50 percent of Americans will be diagnosed with a mental illness or disorder at some point in their lifetime.

- 1 in 5 children, either currently, or at some point during their life, have had a severely debilitating mental illness.

- 1 in 5 Americans will experience a mental illness in a given year.

- 1 in 25 Americans live with a severe mental illness, such as schizophrenia, bipolar disorder, or major depression.

ROOT CAUSE

These three pathways of psychedelic medicine, dreams, and rituals can help us find the root cause of our pain and suffering and a new perspective from which to live. This is not a one-size-fits-all solution—everyone must find their own path and can potentially learn to do so. From my experience counseling people, we have lost touch with time-honored rituals and ceremonies—and even relatively simple things, like connecting with one another on a personal level by sharing our stories. Therefore, so many of us have all sorts of mental health issues that we simply cannot seem to escape. Many seek relief from the pain without getting to the root cause. Some seek to numb the pain with alcohol, shopping, social media, sex, food, gaming, overworking, or other means to simply fill the void and not feel anything at all.

INVESTIGATING THE TRANSPERSONAL
DIMENSIONS OF OURSELVES

These three powerful pathways are a means to connect with the transcendent and transpersonal dimensions of ourselves beyond the limits of our personal identity in the jar. Each pathway allows for the experience of going beyond our ordinary physical universe as we know it and connecting us with our non-ordinary state of consciousness, bringing our whole life together as mind, body, and spirit into focus.

These non-ordinary states can manifest in dreams, rituals, and psychedelics. The three inner pathways allow for connection in the community, a sense of belonging, and a deeper level of relation with one another. Together, these pathways bring the power to transform our consciousness into our own hands. In transforming ourselves, there is a greater potential for transforming the collective consciousness in our world today.

A WOMAN'S VOICE IN PSYCHEDELICS

My practical guidebook is written from a woman's perspective, my wisdom and intuition, my heart, and my own healing journey of transformation. I share my real-world knowledge as one who has taken the three pathways for many years and accompanied others on their healing journeys.

Now, we will join together on this journey. I am grateful you have invited me to be your guide for a short time on these pathways. Then, one day, perhaps you may be a guide for others on their journey.

CREATING THE JOURNEY

The first section of the book is rich, with some fifty pages dedicated to the *Psychedelic Journey Guidebook.* It is for those just starting out, to more advanced and experienced therapists and facilitators who want to add new therapeutic tools to their collection. Included are practical ways for helping to create a good journey, and for keeping it simple yet covering all the protocols for preparation. I have worked in the field of psychology as a therapist for a long time, so these guiding ideas are synthesized from years and years of working with and training others, with simple steps to follow on the path to inner healing.

Partnership with one another is a way to be in the world and socially organized. We can consciously become "co-creators of our own evolution."

This is the vision I hold for us all.

We are co-creators of our own evolution as partners, and there is always room to evolve in our partnerships.

We must understand our collective story, create a new image for a partnership way in the world, speak our truth, and glimpse images of the unitive consciousness that moves us all forward together. It starts by simply knowing and telling our stories. It continues by honoring all our unique journeys as women and men, LGBTQ, black, white, brown, people of all cultures, and all countries of origin embracing the beautiful diversities of human-kind, including all species of creatures and sentient beings that live on this blue-orbed planet Earth together.

THREE INNER PATHWAYS: PSYCHEDELIC MEDICINE

The first inner pathway is through psychedelic medicine, which opens us to multiple dimensions beyond the one we are in now. It offers the experience of glimpsing our existence from a wider lens of perception and creating a potential for mystical openness. Psychedelics provide an initiation into the direct experience of our wholeness or holiness and perhaps touch into numinosity through a non-ordinary state of consciousness. Utilizing psychedelic medicine is similar to entering into the dream realm; only we are awake and lucid.

This is not an altering of consciousness but instead an expansion and increasing consciousness, which opens us to a greater field of reality. We have only begun to scratch the surface of what there is for us to know and understand through psychedelic medicines. There are over thirty million psychedelic users in the United States.

DREAMS

The second inner pathway is through our dream dimension, which takes us to a rich and powerful interior landscape of our being. Dreams are our internal narratives and stories inviting us to talk with central wisdom figures, engage with symbols, receive valuable guidance, understand the archetypal realm, and give us illumination for our life journey. We all dream.

We can discover the experience of dreamwork, joining our present experience with our past, from which we form a relationship of continuity (or a continuing unity) with the wholeness of our lives. Which then integrally connects us to the collective wholeness of all life. The deeper living of our whole life includes transformative dream interpretation, which we will learn, living more mindfully aware and holistically, and seeing ourselves as a whole person living in a world intimately interconnected. Dreams are a pathway into our "holistic" view of ourselves and our world.

RITUALS

The third inner pathway is through our experience with creating fresh rituals and ceremonies and opening ourselves to initiation into new life experiences. Rituals help us to make closure, relieve anxiety, or celebrate a happy occasion. Rituals bring comfort, an awareness of order, and an understanding of meaningful patterns. Rituals and ceremonies also allow us to enter the expanded experience of connection in the community. We enter a sense of what is a powerful, unitive energy, omnipresent, here and now, and connecting us all the time. We have all taken part in rituals during our lifetime where we felt something move collectively through everyone as one unifying experience, during a meditation, drumming circle, music festival, or medicine ceremony. We can use rituals to commemorate what we have learned during our medicine experiences.

In ritual, we can creatively engage in cleansing ceremonies for preparation and release from what comes as revelations and insights offered by our dreams or the medicine experiences. In our relationships, we can imaginatively enter healing rituals to put closure to toxic and unhealthy relationships from the past, where we may have had poor boundaries. Through a variety of inspired rituals and ceremonies, we can make closure using sage, smudging, or burying symbolic objects in the ground and honoring our endings and new beginnings, affirming our rites of passage.

Through rituals, we can initiate ourselves into new life beginnings with baptism in a river, in the ocean, or floating things down little streams. We can experience a more unified and fortified love relationship with rituals and ceremonies in the community. In partnerships, we share rituals of unifying our deepest connection of intimacy with one another through marriages and unions, which celebrate using singing, dancing, taking vows, and playing music in a sacred space.

TRIUNE-THREE-FOLD CORD

Any of these inner pathways, independently, will move us to the experience of our transpersonal and transcendent realm and non-ordinary states. The three intertwined together are strongest for deepest healing and inner transformation. Just as a three-fold cord, I mentioned can withstand a great deal more pressure than a single or double cord. We will tether ourselves together on the inside with the triune cord, combining the integration of dreams, rituals, and psychedelic medicines. Woven together on our journey, the three are mightier than any one pathway taken alone. We are stronger taking this journey in community with one another and having this guidebook in hand.

THE CONNECTION IN THE COMMUNITY OF TRAVELERS

The triune pathway is also about community. We are taking the psychedelic, dream, and ritual journey together. If there is trouble on any one of the pathways, we will prevail and get through it when we travel together. One alone on the psychedelic journey may feel overwhelmed or overpowered. But two can withstand what one cannot do alone, and three together can withstand even more.

The community of travelers on the psychedelic pathway makes an enormous difference. We give attention to who we invite to be on our journey. There is a vulnerability. We are taking the journey together into our interior world, understanding non-ordinary states of consciousness, and valuing our innermost life and transcendent existence. My recommendation is to journey together with a therapist, facilitator, or trusted community of friends. Psychedelic medicine is traditionally a nondirected approach. However, being nondirected does not necessarily mean we are supposed to do this deep inner work alone without any directions, support, or guidance. Always remember, we do better and are safer when we travel together.

TRIUNE PATHWAYS: THREE-FOLD CORD

The triune pathways create a grounding and synergy that will withstand the test of time and be everlasting. Weaving the three-fold cord or inner pathways together fortifies the healing experience. We have the inner validation that sustains the newfound resilience of the lived experience, touching into more dimensions of our being. In touching these multiple dimensions, integrating the inner healing process creates a permanent effect on our lives and daily life experiences. In collaboration, the pathways can bring our deepest wisdom and understanding that becomes an indelible imprint on our psyche. The triune pathway allows the experience of transcending the ordinary and traveling to the mystical dimension within us.

SUFFERING IS A PART OF LIVING

Life is difficult, and suffering from trauma is painful. Once we accept this, we can transcend it because we will not be stuck in the pain and suffering, thinking it will never end and go on forever.

Pain is not assigned to us as something that must be carried daily with its heaviness. This is where much of the day-to-day suffering and heaviness from recurrent depression and anxiety come from. The thought that this emotional suffering will always be a part of the generational family pattern of trauma is difficult to deal with alone.

I have worked with many people who, once discovering that they can let go of their pain, are worried about letting it go because it is so familiar, like an acquaintance, so to speak. If they let it go, who would they be then? How would they feel without the pain? The pain for some has become an old familiar companion. They do not know themselves without the pain. They feel a bit afraid to let the pain go.

When psychedelic medicine helps them see and feel the lightness of not having to carry the pain, they don't immediately know how to adjust or respond to being without the companion of pain. At first, they are amazed, then curious, and some are perplexed by the feeling of being out from under the pain.

FEAR OF FORGETTING THE PAIN

Some veterans with PTSD have described the worry of forgetting the pain. If they somehow forget the pain and suffering, they may not be able to help other veterans with their own pain. This is not an uncommon concern. There is a way to transform and use the experience of being wounded by the pain of trauma. The trauma is a wound and often leaves an emotional scar. Trauma and wounds can heal, but the scars remain as part of the life story. Our scars tell the stories of our lives.

What are we letting go of then? We are letting go of the emotional, mental, psychological, and physiological heaviness and weight of the pain. The heavy pain of trauma can cause ongoing depression and energetic depletion and zapping of our vital life force. The energy drain often happens daily for those who have suffered life traumas.

One man who had long-held depression once said to me during his very first psychedelic session, "Is this lightness the way most people feel all the time?" He was shocked and amazed with his eyes closed outwardly yet wide open inwardly to a new reality and feeling of lightness. He had been trapped in the heaviness of his trauma pain for so long that he did not know what it felt like to have it lifted for a while. I answered, "Yes, for some." I guided him to make a vivid memory of this lightness in his body, mind, and spirit so he could come back to this internal feeling of lightness again and again. This inner healing work is best done with an integrative psychotherapy approach by a trained therapist or facilitator, where we begin to tell the story of our life and witness our journey of healing and transformation together.

Triune
Pathway One:
Psychedelics

Chapter One provides a planned and methodical outline of questions, exercises, journaling prompts, and self-exploration that are meant to help with the presession preparation of how to be on the medicine journey, and then post-integration questions and prompts utilizing rituals and dream work. These are tried-and-true methods that can be used with your clients for facilitation and therapeutic counseling.

Chapter Two describes how psychedelic medicine is an accelerator for openness when used with much gentleness and care. This experience needs to be approached with reverence and awe. It is helpful to see yourself as a midwife for the soul of the person you are working with. Some of the things shared are from some of the best psychedelic teachers in the field, such as Dr. Janis Phelps, and how she approaches getting the most out of the medicine journeys and the rebirthing process.

Origin stories are also a part of Pathway One, and I tell my personal story of my first experience with LSD in **Chapter Three**. In psychedelic circles, there is a tradition of sharing your "origin story," the first experience you had of using a psychedelic substance. Understanding the transforming effects of your first experience with a psychedelic and the non-ordinary state of consciousness can be informative.

1

Psychedelic Journey Guidebook

You are about to go on a trip, a journey into yourself. Using the simple analogy of taking a trip, there may be things you would have prepared and packed for your trip. You would create a checklist of things that are essential to take on your journey depending on where you were going and what you would absolutely need to make it the best trip possible. One carry-on bag will be packed with everything that is vitally important to make the trip successful and make yourself comfortable. Perhaps another checked bag for things, just in case, so you will be prepared for whatever may come up on the trip.

This section is your guidebook to becoming more knowledgeable on how to get packed and ready for your journey. It is a guide to prepare you for the best possible psychedelic journey or trip. This can help by giving you clarity on how to prepare to take the journey and get the most out of the trip.

You would not leave the country without having your passport and knowing the language, currency, etiquette, and social norms. Likewise, this guidebook will give you a better understanding of the land within your own being, the language of your inner world, the currency of the transpersonal landscape, and how to navigate with your inner healer. All of this while having appreciation, grace, and kindness toward yourself on this trip.

You will learn how important it is to have a good personal guide on your journey, preferably a well-trained psychedelic therapist or facilitator. You will learn what to pack in your bags, how to prepare yourself in mind, body, and spirit for the journey and how to have the best psychedelic journey possible.

The following are preparation sections that are in your guide-book; look at each one:

- Pre-Journey Counseling

- Preparation questions for the psychedelic journey

- Plural Beingness--Who is on your bus?

- Inviting your Inner Healer

- Meeting Your Shadow

- Tools to pack in your bag before you go on the trip

- Being present on your journey

- Getting past your ego

- Handling the twists and turns of grief with grace

- Being on the trip and unexpected things that may come up

- Integration following the journey

- Creating an integration mind map and ritual for remembering the trip

- Continuing the inner healing work weeks and months later

EVERY JOURNEY IS DIFFERENT

Every trip you have ever taken in your life is unique and different, even if it is to the same place. Similarly, every psychedelic journey is unique and different. There are no two journeys that will ever be the same for you. Your opportunity is to do all you can to prepare yourself, select the right medicine for your journey, and, most importantly, have the best available therapist or facilitator with you during your trip. Once your preparation is done, you can relax a bit more and know that you are ready to allow, trust, and be the medicine, by flowing with what will be revealed and staying present to the revelations on your journey.

INNER RITE OF PASSAGE

There is a growing movement of people like yourself who thirst for this inner rite of passage. Who have searched outwardly to the external world predominately and have come up empty or found it disappointing. Now ready, you can take the rite of passage into your own internal world, deepening your beingness and have it networked and unified together. You can fulfill your own need for inner-world connection, inner sacred space, visiting your own inmost sanctuary. Perhaps your inner journey and this trip is what you have been searching for all along.

WHAT DOES IT MEAN TO SHIFT BEYOND
YOUR EGO TO YOUR INNER WORLD?

The journey to finding yourself often involves leaving your every-day awareness and entering another dimension of yourself. By doing so you take a journey to novel places, like visiting a foreign land. The inner world for many may seem like a foreign country. As with all hero and shero journeys, there must be a leave-taking, for there to be a homecoming. The hero or shero must leave one aspect of the known self, the ordinary state of consciousness, to enter the unknown dimension of deep self, the non-ordinary state of consciousness. This can be a journey to your inner self, and the origin of your beingness. All of these lie beyond the boundaries of physical matter, beyond space and time, beyond the ego.

HAVING A THERAPIST, COUNSELOR, OR
FACILITATOR JOIN YOU ON YOUR JOURNEY

Your psychedelic journey will be best if you have support. Some experienced travelers on the psychedelic path prefer to do their journey independently. However, you will gain the most out of your experience if you do this with someone who knows how to support you. That support needs to include presessions, prepa-ration, the actual journey, then the post counseling integration sessions with lots of personal introspection work along the way, and after.

INITIATION: THE BEGINNING

Every journey will have a beginning, a middle, and an end. Approaching the journey with openness and curiosity is best. Having a mindset that is referred to as the beginner's mind. Not already trying to predict or analyze what is going to happen. Relaxing personal judgments and seeing your journey as a first-time experience. Even if you have traveled using psychedelic medicines before. Seeing this journey with fresh eyes.

Following, you will find a poem I wrote after completing my master's thesis. My poem reminded me of the chants and the "I am" statements I heard from a wise teacher, Maria Sabina, whom I have dedicated this book to, and you can read about it in the dedication. At the time I authored this poem, I did not know about Maria Sabina. However, I found it interesting that I used the same "I am" phrasing pattern in the healing rituals and ceremonies as she did.

USING POETRY AS A PASSPORT AND INITIATION

You need a passport to leave the country, and poetry is a great passport into your inner world. All journeys begin with initiation and creating a rite of passage. My poem is an initiation for you, a rite of passage into your inner world where your power and pathway to your Inner Healer exist. My suggestion is to read this poem to yourself, or aloud, as a means of marking your beginning, your entrance, or your passport into a new experience of your inner world.

By marking this moment, you are leaving one way of being in the world and welcoming or accepting an invitation to another way of awareness. You are opening yourself to an expanded sense of your own inner transformation or "rebirth." You are acknowledging to your wise and deepest self that you are preparing and entering a relationship with your true self, your authentic self, and the inner vision that will take you there with this poetry passport.

You are leaving the known and inviting the deeper meanings of your existence to come to you, which may be the unknown. Opening to this inner vision reveals your transcendent self, beyond this outer world into the transpersonal and non-ordinary states of consciousness. In this place, access your deepest knowledge and your innate wisdom.

SPIRIT HEALER

By Gay Lynn Grigas

I am power.
I am soul unfolding.
I am the lotus with petals of wisdom opening.
I am the candle that illumines the mind.

I am the sage and fire that cleanses.
I am the drum that beats in rhythm with the heart drum.
I am the resurrection.
I die to the old and celebrate the emergence of the new.

I honor the ancient wisdom of the ages.
I am the communion of all people.
I am the pain of love and the joy of sorrow.
I am honest, reflecting, risking, and sharing.

I am the trust that opens and heals.
I am wholeness.
I am being, belonging, and becoming in expression.
I am the sacred space of ritual.

I am aware.
I am the journey to new places within.
I am, with intention, transcending daily waking conscious.
I am growing, and time and space grow more relative.

I am the mystery.
I am intuitively one with all life, all people.
I am embracing the unity of all that is.
I am the images, the keys to unlocking new worlds.

I am Spirit.
I am energized and alive.
I dance the dance and then let it dance me.
I am breathing, touching, tasting, smelling, hearing.

I am the music of the earth.
I am the peace that is real and eternal.
I am radical aliveness.
I am peaceful death.

I am being.
I am non-being.
I am ageless.
I am order, the progressive movement of the soul upward.

I am the spiral, the alpha and omega.
I am defining and re-defining.
I am the dream that awakens.
I am the surprise.

I am the fear. I am the love.
I am the initiation into new life experiences.
I am the rite-of-passage.

I am the opening to new discovery.
I am the voice of the heart's soul.
I am ritual.
I am Spirit Healer.

PRE-JOURNEY COUNSELING

The presession with psychedelic medicine helps to create a set, or mindset, that simply and literally opens all kinds of doors in our consciousness to our own truth. Remind yourself that you hold the keys to your own freedom. With a bit of curiosity, humility, and willingness, you can free your own imprisoned splendor. You can open to self-love rather than self-loathing. You open to the greater realms and dimensions of your life that are here for you all the time.

PRESESSION INCLUDES:

- Meeting with your therapist or facilitator at least one to three times before the journey. For deepening the experience, meeting three times in advance is preferred.

- Setting up protocols for communication before the first journey to ensure trust and safety.

- Review the flight instructions.

- Navigate the boundaries around touch or no touch.

- How to manage turbulence or other worries and concerns.

- Understanding what it is like being in a non-ordinary state.

- Protocols for entering the experience of non-ordinary states of consciousness.

- Grounding and breathing with meditation practice.

- Allowing for all the parts of yourself.

- Hearing the messages from within for healing.

- Creating a mindset and a harmonious healing setting.

- Coming with openness, curiosity, and humility.

With psychedelic medicine the emphasis is on allowing, letting, and being. Practicing breathing support helps with the grounding when the journey becomes intense. The presession shows you how to have the willingness to be spontaneous and present and is an invitation to all the parts of the self to come forward and feel accepted, allowing for each part to be seen with love and compassion. It is building a trusting container for the work to be done.

Preparing and coming into the journey with a deep and profound reverence for the experience, opening to the opportunity to see and hear from the most voiceless and disenfranchised outcast parts of ourselves, and to let those abandoned parts of the personality know they have a place and a purpose.

PREPARATION FOR PSYCHEDELIC JOURNEY: REFLECTION QUESTIONS BEFORE THE JOURNEY OR RITUAL

During the presessions, take time to journal. You have the following questions to open you to new insights. Use a personal journal with more pages than are available here and explore your personal background and history. Write the following questions before your journey and share them with someone you trust, a therapist or facilitator. Setting goals in advance will help you track your progress.

For the big picture you may have overall goals you would like to achieve, for example, healing from past trauma, addiction, depression, anxiety, or codependency. There have been generational patterns that you have become aware of repeating and now you want to address and heal from these patterns. You may also have life changes you are navigating and need support in making these changes. In the section below name your big goals now:

Three big picture goals you would like to achieve:

1 ....

2 ....

3 ....

EXISTENTIAL QUESTIONS

These are called your existential questions: What is the meaning and purpose of my life? People suffer because they feel that their lives have no existential meaning or purpose, and they feel empty. Before your psychedelic journey, begin to prepare by reflecting on the meaning and purpose of your life. This may be the first time you have ever looked at these bigger life questions. This is okay because you are entering the transpersonal, or beyond personal, sense of your life and existence. Remain open and willing to allow your own beliefs and awareness to appear in your own way.

The next questions are for continuing preparation and will help you to deepen your experience by writing your answers to these bigger life and existential questions. This will help you gain the most insight. Please write and reflect on the following questions. You can write as much or as little as you want. If it is easier to bullet point your answers, that works too.

Who I was?

....

....

....

....

Who I am?

....

....

....

....

Who do I want to be?

....

....

....

....

REFLECTING ON THE BIGGER
EXISTENTIAL LIFE QUESTIONS:

....

You do not have to answer all of these questions, just the ones that help you explore yourself on the inside. Answer the questions to the best of your ability and answer only the questions that best reflect what you would like to understand about yourself. This is not a test or a competition and there are no right or wrong answers. You are simply exploring your thoughts and feelings by creating your own inner-world connections. This is a starting point. Your reflections on your journey up to this point in your life may have been outwardly focused, but now you are looking within and beyond.

Again, this may be the first attempt to journey into your inner world and invite these answers to come to your awareness. Take things slow. Just asking the questions of yourself is enough. Then you will begin to slowly bring things up from your deeper self and allow the responses to surface in your awareness. Remember there are no right or wrong answers. Take this as an inner quest, each question will show you something. Take the pursuit slow and with curiosity and it will open you to new discoveries and learning something interesting about yourself.

What is the meaning of my life?

....

....

....

....

What is the purpose of my life?

....

....

....

....

Am I living true to myself?

....

....

....

....

What motivates me most?

....

....

....

....

What is truly of value to me?

....

....

....

....

What is my truth?

....

....

....

....

MEETING ALL THE PARTS OF YOURSELF ON THE BUS!

Now is your time to have the parts of you come into the light, be seen, and be integrated into your whole self. In any kind of inner work you discover the parts of yourself. Keep present with this process of internal dialogue with the parts of yourself. A helpful visualization to meet all the parts of yourself is to imagine a bus, and on this bus are all the parts of yourself. Remember, all the parts of you on the bus are good. There are no bad parts that get tossed off the bus and rejected. You must look around and see who is on your bus.

- Who is on my metaphoric bus?
- What is their story?
- Where did they originate from, inside of you?

You have numerous parts of yourself. We all do. You can begin to recognize your parts and get to know them. The parts are always with you, and now you can see what they need and how they can work together in partnership with one another.

In our healing and recovery process, we are often recovering parts of the lost self. Author, and Jungian Analyst, Robert Johnson, writes in his book *Ecstasy,* "We like to think of ourselves as individuals. But it is important to remember that, on a deep level, we are *plural beings.* That is, we are one being made up of quite a few distinct personalities, behaviors, and archetypes, all looking for expression. When we first dip beneath the surface in search of these personalities, we may feel insecure because we are in uncharted waters. For this reason, the first appearance of the god can be terrifying, and your first response may be to run for your life. Do not!"

Keep present with this process of internal dialogue with the parts. You have so much more inside you than you may have realized. Now is your time to have the parts of you come and introduce themselves, be invited to speak and tell us who they are and what they need so they can join you on the journey, more fully present as a part of your whole self.

Here are a few suggestions and ideas of the possible parts that may be on your bus and there may be many more:

☐ Child part   ☐ Parent part

☐ Teen part   ☐ Angry or frustrated part

☐ Adult part   ☐ Rebellious part

☐ Stubborn part

☐ Creative part

☐ Family member parts: son, daughter, husband, wife, partner, sister, brother

☐ Achiever part

☐ Lazy part

☐ Sad part

☐ Happy part

☐ Competitive part

☐ Fearful or scared part

☐ Curious part

☐ Shutdown part

☐ Compassionate and loving part

☐ Confident part

☐ Terrified part

☐ Worried part

☐ Friendly part

☐ Isolated part

☐ Wise part

☐ Knowledgeable part

☐ Confused part

☐ Inner Healer or Spiritual, Divine Self part

☐ Resilient part

☐ Self-destructive part

☐ Addict part

☐ Assertive part

☐ Weak or vulnerable part

☐ Honest part

☐ Dishonest part

☐ Entrepreneurial part

☐ Modest part   ☐ Awkward part

☐ Wounded part   ☐ Logical part

☐ Socially conscious part   ☐ Emotional part

Who is on your bus? Add to your own list.

What parts of yourself are on your bus that you can recognize now?

All these parts of yourself are always there. The most important question you need to ask yourself now is:

"WHO IS DRIVING THE BUS?"

What part of you is driving the bus at any time in your day-to-day life? Let this become a new awareness. It could be any part of you at any time that is driving your bus. If the fearful part of you is driving the bus, you know what kind of ride you are going to have. If the angry part is driving, it may be a rough ride, and everybody better buckle up!

1. First thing to work on is becoming aware of the parts of yourself. Who is on your bus?

2. Second, which part of you is driving the bus? Is that the best part of you to have behind the wheel right now?

3. Third, if that is not the best part of you to be driving your bus right now, how can you negotiate to get some other part behind the wheel without crashing the bus or your life?

This is an effortless way to gain some clarity at any given moment. If you are stressed out or depressed and anxious, what part of you is driving? Then begin to have an internal dialogue and hash things out with that part of you. You cannot just ignore that depressed part, you must negotiate with that part of yourself to collaborate and work together with the other parts of you that can help. This begins to build an internal dialogue, a positive self-talk, between the parts. Then internally they are recognized and in a healthier relationship with one another, adding to your emotional maturity and self-awareness, as well as your love and self-compassion.

The Pixar movie, *Inside Out,* did a wonderful job of out-picturing how the emotions named as characters––Joy and Sadness. They had to team up to support one another and collaborate to help the main character navigate a challenging time of emotional growth and change in her young life. You must do the same and understand how the parts of yourself can collaborate and best support one another.

For example, in the movie, Joy wanted to avoid Sadness, but Sadness was an important part of the inner healing process for Joy to fully appear. The theme is finding inner unity within us and welcoming the distinct parts of you is a valuable exploration. The ability to become aware of the various parts of our personality and have them working more collaboratively on the inside.

REMEMBER: THE MOST INTELLIGENT
CONVERSATION YOU MAY HAVE ALL DAY IS THE
ONE YOU ARE HAVING WITH YOURSELF!

Learning how to integrate the parts of yourself before the medicine journey is helpful. You may see parts of yourself differently. There may be parts of you that can help while on the medicine journey. There may be parts of you that show up on your journey and you will have familiarity with them and be able to recognize them. You can have a dialogue with them and negotiate who is going to be driving the bus or driving your journey. For example, if anxiety or control is driving the bus, it is going to be a tougher ride. The part of you that is courageous, exploitative, and curious needs to take the wheel of the bus.

PREPARING FOR THE VULNERABILITY
OF THE PSYCHEDELIC JOURNEY

There is a vulnerability when entering non-ordinary states of consciousness. It is creating a feeling of safety within you and deals with any fears that may come up inside while on the journey. Preparation for the psychedelic journey is really preparing yourself to take a deep dive into your own being. It is not as much a leave-taking as it is an inner homecoming.

Knowing and regularly doing grounding techniques, breathing exercises, mindfulness practices, spiritual activity, personal ritual, and ceremony are important to ready yourself to be on the psychedelic journey.

During the non-ordinary states, a full range of emotions may present themselves, and using a variety of breathing and grounding techniques will help you. The journey with the psychedelics is about moving toward what is there in your mind and spirit. A willingness to be open to what comes forth rather than running or fleeing from it.

The best advice when something starts to frighten or chase you is not to run but to move toward it, face it, and see what it has to say to you. Reaffirming this willingness by saying to yourself "I take the next step and breathe." The various breathing methods can be practiced in advance and will aid you in self-soothing while moving through more difficult phases that sometimes come up during the psychedelic journey.

SIMPLE PHRASES FOR GROUNDING AND CENTERING DURING THE JOURNEY

Sometimes a "phrase" may be used, like a mantra, or affirmation to help you stay in the flow.

Phrases such as:

"Go with the flow."
"Trust and let go."
"I am willing to see what I need to see."
"Open the door."
"What can I learn?"
"I am not alone."
"I am safe I am protected."
"This is what I signed up for."
"I lean into what wants to be revealed."
"Breathe and take the next step."

These are helpful ways to stay open to what is being revealed. Have this phrase, affirmation, or mantra figured out in advance.

What is your grounding phrase or mantra to help you on your journey?

....

....

....

....

YOUR INNER HEALER: INVITING YOUR INNER HEALER

There are many names for this Inner Healer part, including: Divine Self, Buddha Nature, Loving Presence, Higher Power, God and Goddess, Creative Intelligence, Divine Matrix, Universe, Christ Within, and Tao, known by many names, but all the same healing presence of inner beingness that is part of you.

Your inner healing journey is realized when you are open and willing to meet all the parts of yourself. Then you have the possibility of meeting your Inner Healer, which is already a part of your inner world and within you all the time.

You have an Inner Healer right now. But like an old friend you have not seen in an exceptionally long time, you must create the invitation and send the messages in your dreams, enter the ritual and the psychedelic medicine ceremony, and welcome your healing presence. This may be the part of yourself with a capital "S" our highest Self and best Self.

There is a connection needed, a call to be made, and a message to be sent. And ultimately a message to be received. As you open to your inner healing pathways, there is a stream of communications from your Inner Healer to you from your inner world. It takes a willingness to surrender your control, and from having to do things your way.

WRITE AN INVITATION TO YOUR INNER HEALER

Dear Inner Healer,

....

....

....

....

TRUSTING YOUR INNER HEALING INTELLIGENCE

Trusting your inner healing intelligence is part of your preparation for your psychedelic journey. To trust the guides, spiritual teachers, angelic beings, ancestors, and light beings from other dimensions who often show up. To trust the experience to bring forth whatever is needed for your healing and growth. Your part is to trust and follow and not get ahead of the medicine. Let go and release your need to know what is going to happen and not try to direct the journey yourself.

INTENTION AND PERSONAL SET & SETTING PREPARATIONS

Before your psychedelic journey, set your intention. This does not have to be complicated. In fact, keeping it simple is often best. If this is the first time, the intention might be to experience the medicine and what the journey is going to be like for you. If you have taken a journey before, you know what you want to do and have an intention, aim, or plan. Part of the journey is learning to trust, and trusting whatever comes up on the trip may be needed, even if it is not something you fully understand in the moment.

BEGINNING WITH INTENTION

Part of the healing journey with a psychedelic journey can be enhanced by setting an intention.

- The intention may be to let go and fully trust the inner healing intelligence.

- The intention to renew and restore yourself.

- The intention of re-calibration of your inner world and taking the journey of surrender.

- The intention to know deeply the inner workings of your being.

- The intention of choosing love, happiness, and joy while embracing the innocence that prevails within you.

All these intentions plus more are readily available beyond the ordinary state of conscious awareness. Part of your intention may be letting go of your ego and getting out of default mode. This includes your own need to control the outcome. Here is a sample list of things that have been written as intentions.

Look at the list of illustrations to help spark your own intention. Create the mindset you need just for you before entering your sacred journey.

Sample intentions:

- Letting go of my ego identification.

- Letting go of control.

- Only comparing myself to myself.

- Experiencing more of my Inner Healer.

- Getting out of default mode.

- Do I want the problem, or do I want the answer?

- Knowing at this moment I already have what I need.

- If I ask, I will receive.

- Help me see only love and unmask my fear.

- Loving and accepting my body.

- Knowing what it means to be awake and totally one with the Divine.

- Knowing my true identity and home.

- Being in God as God is being in me.

- Healing the fears hidden in my own mind.

- Reconnecting with the parts of myself that are disconnected.

- Moving through my fear of being separate and alone.

- Seeing the big, big picture.

- Integrating my shadow.

- Own my own inner power.

Write intentions for your journey:

If this is your first journey, it may be good to get familiar with the medicine.

....

....

....

....

PREPARING FOR TURBULENCE

Not every journey is going to be euphoric; some trips may be dysphoric, and you may meet some turbulence and rough patches of travel time. There are always things that happen on trips that we did not expect. The best-laid plans can be spoiled by harsh weather, missed connections, and things coming up we did not plan for. When this happens, we must have the courage and grace to move through the experience, staying grounded and knowing this is all part of the trip.

As you are meeting parts of yourself, you may meet parts that are harder to manage and negotiate with. There may be parts that are angry or frustrated and did not want to have any unpleasant parts of the trip happen and now are having a tough time navigating and may be stuck. This is the reason you have an experienced therapist or facilitator to give you support and help you when you feel scared, fearful, or the feeling of being frustrated is taking over. Some of this may also be related to your personal shadow part.

MEETING YOUR SHADOW

Briefly, there is a part of you known as the personal shadow. When you stand out in the sunlight you will cast a shadow behind you. You and I have a shadow. You may remember as a kid trying to see your shadow, and as soon as you quickly turned around it seemed to disappear. Working with the Shadow energy can be like this elusive and hard-to-see part of yourself. Doing personal shadow work, as it is called in psychology, is a part of your healing process.

In 1886, Robert Lewis Stevenson had a highly provocative dream about a man who swallows a powder and changes so much he is almost unrecognizable. The dream became the foundation for the now-famous story, *The Strange Case of Dr. Jekyll and Mr. Hyde.* The kind and caring physician, Doctor Jekyll, helps tend to and heal people. After taking the powder, he becomes the vicious and destructive Mr. Hyde. The Mr. Hyde part is the nighttime self that has negative emotions such as jealousy, lying, greed, anger, rage, shame, lust, resentment, and suicidal and homicidal tendencies. We all have this part of us that is more masked by our daytime self that is more like Doctor Jekyll. This part of your masked self is known in psychology as the shadow, and you may find this part of you to be unexplored territory in you and may remain untamed.

SHADOW PROJECTIONS

Although it is hard to look at the shadow directly, it does show itself in our daily lives. Shadows can be seen in projections unto others. You may project your own exaggerated feelings onto another person. When we say about another person, "I can't believe she would do that! Or "I can't believe he would say that!" It may be your own exaggerated feelings showing up around others that are really a mirror for yourself to see a part of your disowned or shadowed self. It may be a part of you that is underdeveloped, repressed, or unexpressed. Because it is hard to work with your shadow, it is best done with a caring therapist or facilitator who can help you see what is often hidden. This can be immensely powerful because your shadow often has part of your own power. Integrating your shadow can help heal you and tap into your personal empowerment and help to get to know the hidden or repressed part of yourself that may feel excessively guilty. The healing journey is to make space for the blasphemous and the wounded parts.

NOT FEELING GOOD ENOUGH

Sometimes the shadow is hidden until you have uncomfortable feelings of "not being good enough" or of "shame" exposing your wounded parts. Which then may trigger a cascade of other responses like getting angry, shutting down emotionally, and withdrawing from people. This happens so quickly that you may not even know what is happening. Sometimes what may be coming up is childhood trauma.

Sadly, many children have been victimized and these experiences can be scary and confusing. As children are naturally more self-centered, they often think "I must have done something to cause this to happen. It is my fault!" Or they think to themselves, "I was not a good enough girl or a good enough boy and that made mom, dad, caregivers, or grandparents mad or unhappy." This can easily turn into people pleasing, codependency, and living more externalized to placate and appease others.

Sometimes the child thinks the trauma may be their fault and they were bad and deserved to be punished in this way. The internal thoughts and feelings may turn into "If I was good enough this would not have happened to me." There can be a deep-seated fear of being fatally flawed in some way. The feeling that "I am bad." "I am a mistake." "Something is really wrong with me." Instead of, "I made a mistake," as all human beings and children do. The child may have heard from the wounded and traumatized adults around them, things like, "You were a mistake." "You were an oops." "We wish we never had you." The shame of being deeply flawed in some way will expose these scary thoughts of abandonment. The irrational fears and worries surface, that people will not like me, love me, or want to be close to me, or worse, they will leave me, and I will be alone forever. At the same time, more emotions are suppressed and cut off or shut down, and the shadow grows bigger. Unfortunately, this can continue in adult life and cut us off from our power, our passion, our voice, and living to our fullest potential.

Usually, the shadow self-started in childhood when parts of your childhood self were unacceptable to those around you, and they may have been shutting you down. Perhaps you were told to "stop crying or you would get something to cry about." You may have felt threatened in some way with feelings of rejection or abandonment. Perhaps you were told you were "very bad" or a "disappointment" or "you were a mistake" by someone who was supposed to keep you safe and love and protect you.

So, you stopped crying, being angry, or being noisy out of fear of abandonment. Now you may not be able to cry as easily. So, on the journey you may find that you let yourself cry. This may seem hard at first, but gradually you can open yourself up to allow for more of your feelings and sadness to appear.

Perhaps you were told to be quiet, so now you let yourself have a voice because what was repressed wants to be said aloud. Anger was not allowed, so now let yourself feel the heat and energy of the outraged part and allow it to have a safe space to flow and appear without fear of being rejected. Allow yourself to feel the heat of the anger. Allow the energy to flow into your words and your voice and be transformed and used for something more productive.

SHADOW SELF AND NIGHTMARES—BEING COURAGEOUS

Sometimes, the shadow part can look like something scary on the journey. Similarly, this may be how it shows up in your dream life. A nightmare is dealing with your shadow energies. There may be an impulse in your unpleasant dream of being chased by something or someone. In the space of the psychedelic journey, have the courage to face the scary parts. If possible, make the choice to lean into what is chasing you. You can make your own choice in the moment. If you want to get away, then turn in the other direction. If you are ready to go toward the shadow part, make that choice and reclaim your energy. Be curious about what it wants to give to you.

You always have the possibility of turning away and even running, but first, take a breath, and remember this is the work you came to do. You may have been running from this scary shadow part for much of your life. Now it is time to face it and move toward it. This is another good reason to take your trip with an experienced therapist and facilitator while on your psychedelic journey. That person will know how to guide and help you face your shadow part and integrate the energies into your life using psychedelic medicines as a catalyst.

In doing so with someone you trust as a guide you are shining the light on the parts of yourself you think you do not want anybody else to see or that you may be afraid to show. These parts of you are needed and valuable and may be imprisoned or hidden in the basement of your life. One woman described it as a part of her being locked in the basement or underground prison. Her dreams often reflected this basement scene. One man saw himself in underground tunnels all the time. Again, having support through this with a nurturing and supportive therapist and facilitator is vital. Being reassured that these things come up and may seem fearful or overwhelming, but you are not alone, and you have choices you can make to lean in or not. This is your journey.

YOU HAVE THE KEYS TO YOUR FREEDOM

You have the keys to allow yourself out of the fear of facing the scary parts. It is not outside of you; it is within you. The shadow has an enormous amount of energy. You need this energy to live your life, fuel your creativity, and nourish your health and vitality. Without being integrated, the shadow part can ride roughshod over you and others and can take your energy. It really requires a lot of energy to repress shadow parts and shove them down and keep them repressed until there is an unpleasant explosion of negative feelings and words spoken in haste and anger.

Repressed energies can come out prickly like defensiveness, anger, criticism, and frustration. When they are repressed and shoved down, they often become de-pressed energy. This is a source of your feelings of lethargy and de-pression. It is sometimes the shadow energy trapped in the basement of your body, mind, and spirit. Have the courage to face these shadow parts of yourself, transform this energy, and take back your power and your life force from your shadow part.

You are the only one who can do your interior healing work for yourself. To blame others for your pain and shame is not helpful. Take your power back and know you have the ability and responsibility to respond to your shadow part with self-compassion.

Also, you do not want to take on the responsibility for other people's shadows that are in your life. Being overly responsible and blaming yourself is taking on way too much. You do your work to clean up your own backyard, not your neighbor's yard, so stay focused on your own shadow part and your own healing and you will be amazed how the people around you may change or look different to you as your beliefs of yourself are changed. Get out of the blame-shame game; it is too painful for all concerned.

What am I now aware of that may be a part of my Shadow?

....

....

....

....

Have I had nightmares about something scary trying to get me or chase me and I am running away?

....

....

....

....

What are the unpleasant, insecure, or fearful parts of myself I keep hidden from everyone?

....

....

....

....

Did some of these messages from childhood like "don't cry," or "you are bad," get internalized and make me shutdown emotionally?

....

....

....

....

Is some of this shutting down connected to childhood trauma and abuse, and being used as a defense mechanism by creating a wall or hiding behind a wall inside?

....

....

....

....

Do I have feelings of being depressed or unenergetic that may be connected to some of this repression of my shadow part?

....

....

....

....

PREPARATIONS FOR FACING POSSIBLE
SHAME, GUILT, AND FEAR

Most of us may carry some generational shame, guilt, fear, and anxiety. It is the unresolved family scripts and unconscious behaviors that get passed down from generation to generation. It may never change for generations behind you, but you can change it for your generation and the generations ahead of you. Looking at someone in skin-tight clothes and passing judgment on them saying they are cheap. Resenting people who have money. Perhaps seething with anger when you feel cut off in line or on the road and feeling invisible, and maybe entitled. These may not be just your judgments, but thoughts and judgments passed down from past generations. You can acknowledge these thoughts, and heal them for yourself. Then send them back to the past, to the past generations, now that they have been recognized, healed, and transformed in you.

TEASING OUT SHAME

Understanding and teasing out your guilt and shame and what belongs to past generations is a part of the healing process of freeing yourself to live more fully in the present moment. Otherwise, there is a chance of getting trapped in the museum of the past generations by doing the same thing in the same way and expecting a different result. Your life will not change until you change.

Remember, shame and guilt keep you separated from your true self. You must work inside to tease out the tangles of your life. Some of these questions may help you unlock some of the generational patterns that are being unconsciously repeated. For some, the shame and guilt may feel like a cold, wet, and heavy coat that you are having trouble taking off. It may be that heaviness of the coat of shame that is keeping you separated from your true self.

So, for your inner transformation to take place, you must look at the generational guilt and shame and transform it within your own life. Then you can heal this for every generation coming after you as well. A few things that are familiar generational patterns, are around money, body image, sex, addictions, shame, guilt, anger, jealousy, greed, impatience, and compulsivity, just to mention a few.

HERE ARE HELPFUL QUESTIONS:

What are the generational patterns I am noticing?

....

....

....

....

Did I unconsciously take on this shame, guilt, fear, and anxiety? Whose shame, is it?

....

....

....

....

How can I let go of guilt and shame? Can I forgive it back to that past generation and clear the energy, find compassion for them and myself, and have empathy rather than disdain for them and myself?

....
....
....
....

What do I need to do to take off the wet, heavy, cold coat of shame and guilt that may be creating anxiety and fear for me today?

....
....
....
....

WHAT IS TRAUMA?

You may not even realize that you carry trauma from living through distressing events in your own life. You may only recognize it by having lasting emotional responses connected to that event or similar events when you are triggered. You may have experienced something where you felt unsafe, lost your sense of self, or had trouble regulating your own emotions. Maybe this has made it hard for you to maneuver within your relationships and sustain satisfying emotional connections with others. (Please see Adverse Childhood Experiences ACEs test for more information.)

Your trauma may have come in childhood, in your teen years, or as an adult. There are many types of traumas from natural disasters, sexual assault, physical assault, the sudden death of a loved one, PTSD from active-duty military combat, and first responders' traumas, or being the wittiness of any form of violence being done to another person. One of the most common forms of trauma is emotional abuse, which causes bruises on the inside and can be easily hidden or go unrecognized.

THREE TYPES OF TRAUMAS

There are three main types of traumas: acute, chronic, or complex. Acute trauma may be a result of one single incident. Chronic trauma is repeated and prolonged over a period of time, like childhood abuse or domestic violence. Complex trauma is exposure to multiple traumatic events that are varied and, very disruptive and invasive to your life.

Remember the jar analogy? When you are inside your own metaphoric trauma jar, it is hard to see it more objectively because you are in it. The psychedelic medicine will help you to hopefully come out of the jar and see the jar from the outside, and perhaps see the trauma from a distinct perspective.

Looking at the trauma from outside of the jar gives you a new way to heal and have self-compassion and self-forgiveness. Perhaps seeing things in a way you have never seen before. This can happen just by being able to step back, take a breath, and see yourself from a much broader perspective.

HAVE INFORMED TRAUMA CARE

This is another particularly good reason to have a therapist or facilitator that knows how to collaborate with you and with your trauma. So when it comes up, you are not feeling alone, abandoned, or overwhelmed by having to face your trauma by yourself. You must give yourself permission to have the comfort and support you need to heal your wounds. You would not try to set your own broken leg or remove your own appendix if it ruptured. Do not try to go it all alone and fix all your own trauma. Welcome a trauma-informed therapist or facilitator by your side for support on your journey.

NOTE TO THERAPIST OR FACILITATOR:

If you are a therapist or facilitator, make sure you have done your own trauma work because it may come up, and it can be triggering for you while helping another person in their psychedelic journey. Be prepared by doing your own trauma healing, shadow work, and generational healing of shame and guilt.

Doing your own inner healing work will keep you and your clients safe from transference and countertransference. And if these terms are new to you, do some further reading and exploration. Your role as a therapist and facilitator is to hold the space and container for the healing to happen. The psychedelic work can become very intense at times. If the person you are with is triggered and you are triggered at the same time it can get very messy. Be prepared by doing your own trauma work in advance.

Are you aware of the trauma that has happened to you in your life?

....

....

....

....

Is there a part of this trauma that is getting in your way of living and loving fully and freely?

....
....
....
....

If you could work to heal some of this trauma how would your life and relationships be different?

....
....
....
....

Are you curious to see your trauma from outside the metaphoric trauma jar and gain a new perspective? What do you think you might see differently?

....
....
....
....

Do you know what your triggers are? Such as shutting down, lashing out, being in a fight, fight, freeze, fawn, or faint mode?

....
....
....
....

Can you allow yourself to receive the comfort and support you
need to do your inner healing work?

....

....

....

....

SOMATIC TECHNIQUES

You may hear about somatic work relating to the body, especially
as distinct from the mind. The word somatic is from the Latin
word, soma, "the body." Often, the body holds the memories of
past traumas and events. The body's memories and sensations are
part of your life experience. The somatic techniques that follow
will help you learn to calm yourself or alleviate some of the stress,
tension, and trauma responses that may come up in your body.
These techniques are important for you to practice in advance of
the psychedelic medicine session and include breathing exercises,
mindfulness, meditation, and using the five senses for grounding
and centering. These techniques will help you effectively calm
your nervous system, which may be overloaded or burdened by
stress and reactions to trauma the body is holding.

SETTING UP BOUNDARIES FOR TOUCH

All touch, if it is to be included at all, is agreed upon in advance
in a combination of using mindfulness and breathing with your
eyes closed so that the experience closely resembles the way the
psychedelic medicine session may take place with eyes closed.
A practice session before the medicine session will help set up

healthy boundaries for everyone. Practice all of these before your first medicine journey.

TOOLS TO USE BEFORE YOUR PSYCHEDELIC TRIP

Packing your carry-on bag with these tools before your trip is essential. You will need these on your trip. So, let's get them organized now and begin to know how each of these is essential for a good journey. Practicing these in advance will make your trip so much more pleasant.

- Breathing Techniques
- Mindfulness
- Meditation
- Using the five senses for grounding and centering
- Visual imagery

For those new to meditation, here are the basic seven steps of meditation. Practice for five to ten minutes daily.

1. Sit upright comfortably.
2. Breathe deeply from your navel.
3. Gently close your eyes.
4. Scan your body slowly and notice any tension or sensations.
5. Be aware of any thoughts you are having.
6. When your mind wanders come back to your breathing.
7. Gently open your eyes when you are ready.

UNDERSTANDING MINDFULNESS MEDITATION

Jon Kabat-Zinn—a leader in the field of mindfulness and health—has defined mindfulness as "paying attention in a particular way: on purpose, in the present moment, and non-judgmentally." Mindfulness and thinking in this way are allowing your thoughts to come and go. The more you try to control them, the more invasive they will become. Like your senses, thoughts are a normal part of your existence.

Acknowledge your thoughts and let them pass naturally. You can use the imagery of an open window and let your thoughts blow gently through your mind like a breeze blows through an open window.

Focus on your breathing. Take full but gentle breaths through your nose and notice the rise and fall of your belly. Notice how your body changes as air enters and then leaves your lungs. This is the key to mindfulness meditation. Focusing on the sensation of your breathing will quickly bring you into the present and connect your mind with your body.

PRACTICE BEFORE THE JOURNEY: FOLLOWING
DEEP BREATHING TECHNIQUES

Deep breathing is a simple technique that's excellent for managing emotions. Not only is deep breathing effective, it's also discreet and easy to use at any time or place. Breathe in through your nose, deeply enough that your hand on your abdomen goes up and down, hold the air in your lungs, then exhale slowly through your mouth. Exhale very slowly, this is important. Then time the breathing in this way:

Inhale 1-2-3-4

Pause 1-2-3-4

Exhalation 1-2-3-4

Practice this cycle of breathing for three to five minutes.

Breathing is especially important because there may be times on the psychedelic journey when your breathing rate increases--this is normal. It is extremely helpful not to let your breathing become too fast and then cause you to hyperventilate and trigger overly anxious feelings.

So to safeguard and to help with this intensity, you need to be able to focus on your breathing and stay with one breath, one thought, one moment at a time. Practice this daily in preparation for your journey. Practice with your therapist and facilitator; you will be glad you did.

WAYS OF SELF-SOOTHING FOR GROUNDING

Imagine your safe place vividly. Another valuable idea to keep you in the flow of your journey is to have a few ways worked out ahead of time that you can use to soothe and calm yourself. Doing these in advance can help you easily come back to this calm and centered place inside your mind, body, and imagination. If your journey gets a bit challenging, it is helpful to come back to these thoughts by remembering a time when you were calm and remembering a place that made you feel calm. Practice this in your imagination and use it regularly. Share this with your therapist or facilitator in advance so it can be accessed and resourced quickly.

CREATING A SAFE PLACE IN YOUR IMAGINATION

Create a safe place in your mind and imagine the mountains, forest, ocean, or your home where you feel the most safe and calm. Picture it in detail and practice going there when you become distressed in your day-to-day life. While on the psychedelic journey, this place can be your safe place inside you to return when needed. A woman had a safe place with her grandmother, and she could smell the baking of apple pie and the joy, peace, and calmness of being there with her grandmother. This powerful use of your imagination is very calming and soothing while on the journey.

VISUAL IMAGERY: LETTING GO OF
THE OVERSTUFFED LUGGAGE

Sometimes you pack too much for your trip, your luggage is too stuffed and too overpacked, and you need to lighten the load and pare down what you are taking on your trip. Visual imagery can help you let go of what is the excess baggage you are carrying mentally and emotionally. You want to take just enough luggage to carry the essentials but leave the excess baggage behind. This can be a negative or overstuffed mindset. Go through and sort out what is weighing you down. What is not needed on this trip? Worry, control, overthinking, and fear are just a few things that will weigh you down on any trip.

Your thoughts have the power to change how you feel. If you think of something sad, it's likely you'll start to feel sad. The opposite is also true: When you think of something calming, you feel relaxed. The imagery technique harnesses your power to reduce your anxiety.

DAILY SENSORY TIPS FOR CALMING
AND GROUNDING PRACTICE:

Sounds: Listening to or playing music, soothing voices, nature sounds.

Smells: Aromatherapy or a relaxing bath, a walk in a wooded area, light a candle, bake cookies.

Sights: Spending time outdoors, decorating your space.

Tastes: Eating your favorite food, mint, a good cup of coffee, hard candy.

Activity: A positive, absorbing activity: arts & crafts, attending a performance, guided imagery, playing an instrument.

Questions for grounding, using the five senses:

Sight:
What do you see around you?
What do you notice in the distance?
Look all around to take in all your surroundings.
Look for intricate details you would usually miss.

Sounds:
What sounds can you hear?
Are they soft or loud?
Listen closely to everything around you.

Keep listening to see if you notice any distant sounds.

Taste:
Are you eating or drinking something enjoyable?
What is the flavor like?
How does it taste?
Savor all the tastes of the food or drink.

Feel:
What can you feel?
What is the temperature like?
Think of how the air feels on your skin, and how your clothes feel on your body.
Soak in all these sensations.

Smell:
What scents are present? Are they strong or faint?
What does the air smell like?
Take some time to appreciate the scents.

SETTING: CREATING SACRED SPACE

Creating sacred space is easy when you remember to feed your senses. Remembering the intersections of the sensual and the sacred are important. Each complements one another. Do this with your therapist or facilitator and create the space that makes you feel most relaxed. Your lighting can be bright or dim. Candles can be lit, but there can be more battery-operated candles if that is better. You can ring a bell or chime to begin and end the session. You can start with a poem, phrase, affirmation, or prayer. Choose your favorite scent. Bring something from home, like a picture or object to have with you on your trip. If you like flowers, bring flowers or a single rose.

ENHANCED LIGHTING

Lighting is important and can create a welcoming ambiance in the space of a ritual, ceremony, or your psychedelic journey. Candles are a straightforward way to open the sacred space in the beginning by lighting them and then simply extinguishing them at the end to close the ritual, ceremony, or journey.

ENHANCING AROMA OR SMELL

Smell is important. Choose your favorite scent that is calming and soothing. Remember to speak up if you are sensitive to incense, sage, or other smudging items. Know what smells you like and do not like and ask for these in advance. If you are allergic to anything like perfume or cologne, please let this be known.

SETTING UP AN ALTAR

An altar can be set up as a symbol of a sacred space. Items for the ritual, ceremony, and your journey are placed on your altar. Flowers and things from nature, shells, crystals, and fruits, all can be added.

Place pictures and your own personal items on your altar. If you are doing this with a community of people, you can create an altar together. This can be a community-building and a bonding experience.. Share what you brought and why it is important.

MUSIC SELECTION

The music is a vibrant part of any ritual, ceremony, and journey, so choose a playlist that will best complement the experience. Live music and dance are a glorious part of the ceremony and simple rhythm instruments can be added for interactive joy-making. What would make you most comfortable within a setting:

Smell or aroma:

Music (Best to be instrumental only):

Lighting:

Comfortable Position: Sitting, reclining, or laying:

What are three specific somatic techniques you will use to practice supporting your medicine journey?

1

2

3

Before the medicine journey, all agreements on therapeutic touch must be agreed upon in advance with the therapist or facilitator. It is perfectly okay if you do not want to be touched at all. However, if you think you may need or want a handhold, please be clear and allow this to be in writing.

What agreements with therapeutic touch do I want to make before my medicine session? What is, okay? Be specific.

....

....

....

....

MINDSET

You have been preparing for your journey. You know how to set your intentions. You have prepared yourself to do some of your trauma and shadow work if things come up on the trip. Now, there is one more part that can be a bit challenging. It is like getting through TSA security or customs in the international airport to get access to a new country.

The whole trip and journey can come down to a slow trickle, single file line when you are trying to get past your ego. You have done all this preparation work, planning, getting everything packed, and the TSA Ego Agent says, "Wait! I am not sure you are going to get past me!"

The ego is the controlling part that wants to inspect everything before there is permission to get on that flight. The ego is suspicious. The ego is the hyper-vigilant part that can try to block the departure or at least slow it down.

The TSA Ego Agent may say things and make it hard to leave, making it challenging to go on the journey. It sounds like a negative and critical mindset, saying things like:

"This whole trip is a very bad idea!"
"You should not go. Turn back now!"
"This is crazy."
"Dreadful things could happen!"
"What are you thinking, this is dangerous."
"Leaving the country, leaving yourself, this could be too risky!"

The ego could even say, "You could die!!" The interesting thing is this is true for your ego. It will have grief, experience loss, and lose its tight grip and control of your life. It is very reluctant to let go of the seat of control it has over you. Getting past the TSA Ego Agent is tricky sometimes. However, you are wiser than that part and have been getting ready for this trip for some time now. You are with a good guide, and you can navigate this journey with patience and persistence.

THE CHALLENGE OF GETTING PAST THE EGO

The journey inward is embracing creative ways of understanding yourself and welcoming your true self, your Inner Healer, to join you more fully on your journey to hopefully a better version of yourself using the medicine as a catalyst. Your ego can be looked at as part of your false self. You are not your ego, and your ego is not you. You and I have an existence beyond the ego, sometimes called the impostor self, that only lets in a ridiculously small bandwidth of life and reality. Just like the negative mindset and fear getting through the TSA Ego Agent, be ready to declare your truth without fear and make that passage into a new sense of your true self on your journey. Your ego is not running the show, you are.

Now you can view your beliefs and see them beyond the narrow threshold of the ego. You shift away from being handed or given your belief system and being told what to accept and what to believe, to a fuller understanding of what is true and meaningful for you and your life. Getting to this place of openness can be a challenge. Be patient. You can navigate this part; you are ready. What are some of the last-minute fears or worries that may be coming up for you and your ego?

What do you fear about ego dissolution?

....

....

....

....

How would you deal with your fears of letting go of who you think you are on the journey?

....

....

....

....

Can you let yourself relax and surrender into the observation of yourself beyond your ego?

....

....

....

....

GRIEF AND LOSS EMERGES AT TIMES

Collaborating with your Inner Healer and taking this deep dive within yourself can also bring up feelings of sadness and grief. When this happens, go with what presents itself; there is no right or wrong way to grieve or be on the journey. There are some basic stages of grief and loss that have been named by Dr. Kubler-Ross. These five stages emerge after the death of a loved one, or loss, or major life change.

DENIAL, ANGER, BARGAINING, DEPRESSION, AND ACCEPTANCE

These five stages can appear when there is an experience of unresolved grief following the death of someone, a big life transition, or following any traumatic life event. These stages do not happen in a nice, neat order. Additionally, some of the stages can repeat themselves over time. For example, just when you think you are over the anger, it pops up again.

When you allow your ego to surrender and open to the essence of the Inner Healer within, you can awaken the wisdom within. Through this wisdom, you will be able to walk through these stages of grief with as much humility and grace as possible. The following questions may help:

What is a grief or loss that I am dealing with in my life?

....

....

....

....

Am I aware of the stage of grief I may be in right now?

....

....

....

....

How can I allow for the wisdom of this grief and loss to be my teacher? What, if anything, is it teaching me?

....

....

....

....

What parts of myself can help the grief-laden parts of me that are in pain?

....

....

....

....

Finally ready for takeoff!!

FINAL FLIGHT INSTRUCTIONS:

You are ready to leave. Excellent job on all the planning, packing, and preparing. You are finally ready to take off!

- Remember, you will come back.

- You can lean in and trust the process.

- You can trust your inner healer, your therapist or facilitator relationship, and the medicine.

- This is your trip, and you are in charge, so be curious.

- Perhaps think of yourself as a scientist or an archaeologist exploring new dimensions of your own being.

- Sometimes your body will want to release or make sounds or move; let it happen.

- You can trust your inner healer will not bring you more than you can handle, so relax.

- When something beautiful or magical happens, watch it, explore it, and connect with it.

- If there is something challenging, ask what it is for and be curious. Thank it for sharing.

- If there is a door, open it if you want to.

- If there are stairs, go up or down.

- If you see planets in space, explore them.

- Sense that the music is carrying you, holding you, making a safe place to lean into and breathe. Let the music guide you.

- Be okay with extended periods of silence.

- If you need a light touch or handhold, ask for it.

- If you need physical support, encouragement, or grounding, ask for it.

- You get to say what feels right, you are leading the way.

- Listen, then listen more deeply.

Enjoy the Journey!!

INTEGRATION WORK FOLLOWING THE JOURNEY

Integration is the process of digesting an experience: Identifying and absorbing insights and the newfound wisdom to reveal and support you in becoming your whole and authentic self. Non-ordinary states have the possibility to show you what it is like to be free, expressive, confident, open, and a being capable of love.

These non-ordinary states may also walk you through the ways you are cut off from thriving: fear, isolation, anger, resistance, rigidity, and wounding. Whether positive or negative, a deep experience offers rich insight and guidance for reaching and keeping your wellness.

The following questions are intended to help you make conscious space for the integration of your experience. Time for your personal reflection is a precious gift you give yourself. This intimate act with yourself allows for connecting to your own experience, free from distraction. Honor what is true for you in the present moment, seeing any tendencies to change, deny, or minimize.

Here are the topics for the following questions that will touch on what you may have experienced. Only answer the questions that are important to you and resonate with your personal journey. The questions are prompts to help you explore your journey and remember what may have been important, inspiring, or healing. If there are questions that do not make sense, skip over them. These are the themes to the following questions:

- Thoughts, memories, and reflections on the journey.

- Reflection on your intentions.

- Self-compassion and love.

- Reflections on the transpersonal experience.

- Guides and teachers that showed up.

- Themes, people who came, voices heard, messages received.

- Grief or sadness that came up.

- Inner wisdom figures who came.

- Pathways that may have opened.

- Understanding yourself better.

DRAWING: FOLLOWING THE JOURNEY
USING THE MIND MAP:

A Mind Map uses a tree, or circles, or geometric shapes to represent a brief picture or overview of what occurred on your journey. Do this with your therapist or facilitator. Themes, people, and voices may have come up, briefly capture those right after, if possible, for deeper integration later.

USE THE MIND MAP WHILE ANSWERING
THESE QUESTIONS:

Themes on the journey?

....

....

....

....

Who came to you on the journey?

....

....

....

....

What voices did you hear on the journey?

....

....

....

....

Parts of yourself that showed up?

....
....
....
....

What emotions or energies were repressed or depressed?

....
....
....
....

What anxieties popped up?

....
....
....
....

Were you in the past? Present? Future?

....
....
....
....

Were you aware of any grief or sadness? What are you grieving?

....
....
....

What came to you that may need to be released?

....

....

....

....

Did any Inner Wisdom figures show up?

....

....

....

....

What were their messages for you?

....

....

....

....

Were there any experiences that were frightening?

....

....

....

....

Were there any themes such as death and rebirth?

....

....

....

....

Did you have any experience of feeling connected or belonging?

....

....

....

....

Were there people, places, or things you have never seen before?

....

....

....

....

What pathways opened to you?

....

....

....

....

Were there any new invitations for your healing or growth?

....

....

....

....

Did you sense any new opening to your powers or your passions?

....

....

....

....

*Were there any new neuron-network connections you felt in
your own mind, like an internet superhighway or a download
of added information?*

....

....

....

....

Did you notice any new spiritual connections?

....

....

....

....

*Was there an understanding that your humanity and divinity--
your mind, body, spirit-being, more intricately connected?*

....

....

....

....

*Was there an awareness of the masculine and the feminine, the
yin and the yang within you?*

....

....

....

....

Was there anything that was totally unexpected that happened?

....

....

....

....

These reflection memories, thoughts, feelings, and insights can be written about in the days and weeks to come. The more you write, the more will be revealed.

During the experience did you have life memories, thoughts, or feelings that came up, which have shaped who you are?

....

....

....

....

List a few of your most important memories, thoughts, and feelings.

....

....

....

....

What did they mean to you?

....

....

....

....

What did they inform you about how you have been living?

....

....

....

....

How will these insights be manifested in your life and daily living from now on?

....

....

....

....

List the new awareness that is significant and meaningful to you and that you always want to remember.

....

....

....

....

REFLECTION ON YOUR INTENTION

Remember your intention for this inner healing work.

How did your experience reinforce the direction that you want to go and align with your intention?

....

....

....

....

Are there ways of being, or things that you are doing or not doing, that can support you in your intention?

....

....

....

....

What takes you away from your life purpose or intention?

....

....

....

....

What brings you closer?

....

....

....

....

What will you continue doing or start doing in your daily life that is connected to your life purpose and intention?

....

....

....

....

SELF-COMPASSION AND LOVE

What did you notice about yourself, what did you feel, did you experience a sense of love?

....
....
....
....

How does love want to show up in your life?

....
....
....
....

Are you able to give and receive love?

....
....
....
....

What did you learn or understand about self-love? Self-Compassion?

....
....
....
....

How do you want to relate to and cultivate love in
your relationships?

....
....
....
....

REFLECTION ON TRANSPERSONAL EXPERIENCE

....

If your sense of identity extended beyond yourself to encompass
aspects of the cosmos or universe, or the oceanic oneness of
nature of life beyond matter, reflect on these questions:

What was the most significant insight you had, seeing yourself as
a part of the universe or cosmos?

....
....
....
....

How did this transpersonal and universal view change or deepen
your views?

....
....
....
....

What does it mean for you to be a part of the whole of nature and how does that affect the way you choose to live your life from now on?

....

....

....

....

CREATE AN INTEGRATION RITUAL
FOLLOWING YOUR JOURNEY

The process of doing a ritual will mark your journey completed. You prepared yourself, packed your luggage, left what you knew as your normal state of awareness, and went into a non-ordinary state of awareness on your trip. You returned from the trip and now have new ways to perceive yourself, your life, your meaning of yourself, and your existence.

Now, being back from your journey, you will create a small but significant point of reference by doing a ritual or ceremony to acknowledge the end of your trip. You may choose to take other trips, but this one is over. And now, creating a small ceremony is a way to mark your return. The following are fun and creative ways you can perform a ritual for yourself and include your therapist or facilitator if you like. There are specific rituals and ceremonies created at the end of this book that you can use for reference or do yourself.

THREE STAGES: RITES OF PASSAGE RITUALS

These are the basic ways to think of the stages or parts of a ritual. Use them as a guideline for creating your own ritual and capturing the essence of your trip.

1. Separation or ending ordinary state of consciousness.

2. Transition or entering a non-ordinary state of consciousness when we are neither the old nor the new.

3. Integration or beginning as we move into a new phase, new awareness, new beingness, and synthesis.

When planning a ritual or rite of passage for yourself or someone else, remember these three stages and incorporate them creatively.

HOW WILL I CREATE MY OWN RITUAL AND RITE OF PASSAGE TO HONOR MY JOURNEY?

Create my plan for an integration ritual.

Where will it be?

....

....

....

....

What items will you use?

....

....

....

....

Are there any elements like water, fire, or earth involved?

....

....

....

....

Are you burning something? Are you burying something?

....

....

....

....

Are you planting something?

....

....

....

....

*Are you writing something to honor new insights, letters,
poems, or stories?*

....

....

....

....

Are you using water: lake, stream, or the ocean to cleanse, christen, baptize, or bathe yourself?

....

....

....

....

What can you make to honor and mark your own personal rite of passage?

....

....

....

....

Weeks and Months Following Your Journey

FOLLOWING AND CAPTURING YOUR PSYCHEDELIC JOURNEY:

....

1. Keep a Personal Journal

Focus on the issue that most concerns you currently. Write down thoughts and feelings and ask yourself, "What do I long for?" Transformation can come by actively taking part in your life, acknowledging the quest for deeper meaning, and finding nourishment and support from inner healing resources. Honor your life and your progress by reading over your journal periodically.

2. Complement with the right environment

Each ritual, ceremony, and psychedelic journey has an intention or focus and some required materials. Choose a time and place that is quiet and free from distractions. You may want to honor the sacred space you are creating with a special prayer, incense, music, song, lighting, clothing, candles, pictures, chimes, or other personal means of creating a beginning and end. Be creative; make it an adventure.

3. Keep track of your progress

After you have completed a ritual, ceremony, or psychedelic journey, go back to your journal and write briefly about any awareness, insights, shifts in feelings, changes in mood, or bodily sensations. You may choose to share some insights with a trusted friend, therapist, counselor, facilitator, or a psychedelic support group.

4. Set aside time for play

As new growth and insight take place in your life, relax the intense inner focus. Allow the unfolding of new awareness to take place within. Reach out to others and volunteer or help someone you know in a way that is meaningful to you. Take time to play and be in nature.

5. As you meet blocks (and we all do)

We often shape our lives to avoid what we fear most. Within that fear is all the power you need to change and grow. Through journal writing, discover what is molding and shaping your life. Take charge and confront your fears. By doing so you will gain an enormous sense of power and ability over your own destiny.

6. Celebrate your new growth

Mark your change and new insight with a ritual or ceremony. Celebrate your freedom in living. Author a poem, paint a picture, dance, sing, invite others to a ceremonial dinner. Celebrate your life as a masterpiece in progress.

YOUR INTEGRATION WORK CONTINUES

Keep your dream journal next to your bed every night. Write down all your dreams, even fragments can be helpful.

DREAMS AND PSYCHEDELICS

When working with psychedelics it often crosses the pathway into your dream life and shows you things through visions and your dreams.

Part of the integration work in dream and in the psychedelic journey, is to begin understanding what the dreams or visions on your journey are saying.

Remember that dreams and archetypal images and stories speak a language all their own. They are a symbolic language, not a literal language. Become aware of the symbolic meaning and interpretation for you.

When doing the integration work following a dream, the process is similar.

IT IS BEST TO ASK:

What does this person in your dreams mean to you?

....

....

....

....

What do these symbols, characters, images, and scenes mean to you and how do they relate to your life?

....

....

....

....

This may not be pointing to something happening right away, it is the big picture. Take it for the broader picture of your life journey. This is why the suggestion is made before the journey to not quit your job or leave your relationship right away--if at all, once following a journey. This is an error some people can make. Remember this is a bigger picture you may be seeing that is not happening right now.

TO BE ALIVE IN YOUR OWN EXISTENCE

It is your choice regarding the level and depth of participation in your life experience. On your personal journey, it may have taken you many years to come to the place where you are today. However, there is so much more for you. Work diligently on your dreams and writing in your journal to really begin to feel yourself having a deep relationship with your own existence and taking part in your own life.

Your participation is getting to know yourself beyond the roles by which you normally define yourself, such as family, work, and relationships with others. Ritual, ceremony, dream work, and the responsible use of psychedelic medicine can help in a unique way to explore the terrain of your own life and let the awareness of your own uniqueness appear. You will touch more deeply into your inner healing intelligence. Working with psychedelic medicine can have that indelible impact. You will be opening yourself to your life and existence at greater dimensions and truly be alive and feel connected to all people in a unitive awareness.

THE UNITIVE EXPERIENCE

This unitive experience and awareness is a connectedness that is always present yet often unperceived. The energetic field beyond the personal, leads to peak experiences of the transpersonal, whether in rituals, psychedelic journeys, psychedelic medicine, prayer and healing ceremonies, drumming, or circle work in small communities. All these connective, unitive experiences can have many benefits, as described by leading to a sense of actualizing more of oneself in the oceanic oneness and allness of community and novel realties.

Were you able to touch into the unitive consciousness?

....

....

....

....

How might this help you actualize more of yourself?

....

....

....

....

How do you hold yourself out of the unitive consciousness?

....

....

....

....

How can you open yourself to the allness of community?

....

....

....

....

Do you have an ancestral connection?

....

....

....

....

How were you connected to your own culture?

....

....

....

....

Are there meaningful patterns of your experience and novel realities that you see now?

....

....

....

....

Are you sensing your own belonging and honoring your community and connections?

....

....

....

....

WE END WHERE WE BEGIN

Read the Spirit Healer poem from the beginning again and see how the poem speaks to you about allowing the messages to appear. The psychedelic medicine journey, dreams, and rituals are often more right brain than left brain, and intuitive in nature. The experience is more yin than yang, more allowing and inviting, more being, letting go, and deeply listening. It is a reminder to let psychedelic medicine take us on the journey. Read it again and then write your own "I am" statements.

Write your own "I am" statements:

I am ....

I am ....

I am ....

I am ....

I am ....

I am ....

TIPS FOR SUCCESS

- Work with an experienced psychedelic therapist or knowledgeable facilitator.

- Write in your journal daily.

- Keep a dream journal by your bed and write dreams down every morning

- Read or listen to all the books and podcasts you can on psychedelic-assisted psychotherapy and how it helps with trauma, shame, guilt, codependency, addiction, depression, anxiety, and existential distress. Knowledge is power. Give yourself the power.

- Create your own unique rituals to do your inner healing work and openness to novel realities.

2

Psychedelic Medicine Journeys

MIDWIFE OF THE SOUL

As a therapist or facilitator of the psychedelic medicine journey, think of yourself as a midwife to the soul of the person you are supporting, helping them move through the contractions and pain of their journey. The caring presence of another is important for loving attachment in the most healing manner. Gently remind the person that it is okay to let go and breathe through each contraction and not to resist or become tense or fearful. We know when we resist what wants to come out it may intensify the pain or feeling of being out of control, just allowing what wants to come, to emerge, letting it be birthed.

PSYCHEDELIC MEDICINE IS THE CATALYST

During the journey with psychedelic medicine, there is not a lot to do as you would in traditional therapy. It is a lot of sitting and waiting and listening. That is why the role is sometimes called "Sitter" or "Attendant" and it is quite a different flow than traditional therapy. The medicine is the catalyst for the openness and the receptivity. Some people say, "The medicine did this," or "The medicine said that" which is not exactly the case either, the medicine saying or doing something, other than being a catalyst and an accelerator. It may feel like this at times because in a sense the medicine is an opening of a space within us where we learn about who we really are on the inside. So, it feels like medicine is doing it, but really, we are releasing ourselves into knowing our splendor and magnificence from within our very being. It is an amazing journey within as we close our eyes and remember who we are.

THROTTLE OF OPENNESS

The psychedelic medicine is presenting the opportunity for what wants to emerge from within. It is the throttle for an openness for whatever wants to come up or needs to be revealed from inside us. It is opening a valve, in a sense that would normally reduce so much of life from our awareness. The inner healing intelligence reveals itself much like a dream experience, where you are fully aware, and images symbols and stories are flowing across the screen of the mind.

Psychedelic medicine is a lubricant for the therapeutic process to emerge. Psychedelics, dreams, and rituals are pathways to open us to our inner healing. Our medicine, our inner healing, is already inside of us. The openness and willingness to understand this perception is an important view of the healing process. We come to know that *we are our own best medicine*. We are learning through ingesting the substance how to *be the medicine* for ourselves and one another.

The substance helps as a lubricant with the purging of pent-up emotional tensions, frustrations, anger, or sadness, and by doing so can help in relieving anxiety, depression, and PTSD.

There are three different ways to view what psychedelics can possibly do and how they can work.

The empathogens open the heart and the emotional connection and communion with others:
Example-MDMA

The non-specific amplifiers can reveal aspects of our own mind, conscious, and subconscious:
Example-Ketamine

The entheogens open the pathways of encouraging spiritual connection and oneness:
Examples-psilocybin mushrooms, ayahuasca, and LSD

Huston Smith wrote, "Entheogens is the appropriate word for mind-changing substance when they are taken sacramentally." It is the intention of healing and gaining our own deeper wisdom that is the key.

SACRED WITNESS: THERAPEUTIC AND FACILITATOR SUPPORT

Care is taken to allow the process to unfold. As new perceptions and realities are revealed, some thoughts may be written down by the therapist or facilitator in brief notes in a non-intrusive manner. The facilitator or the therapist is the sacred witness and sometimes the comforter, giving lots of reassurance that the participant is not alone.

LEADER IN THE FIELD OF PSYCHEDELIC-
THERAPY TRAINING

The Center for Psychedelic-Therapy & Research is led by Professor Janis Phelps, PhD. I had the honor and privilege to have a full-day workshop with Dr. Phelps at the International Conference on Psychedelic Research (ICPR) pre-conference training in 2022. Dr. Phelps is a leader in the field of psychedelic therapy training and is the Director of the Center for Psychedelic Therapies and Research at the California Institute of Integral Studies.

As the center's founder, Dr. Phelps developed and launched the first university accredited post-graduate training program for psychedelic-therapy and research. Dr. Phelps 2017 publication, *Developing Guidelines and Competencies for the Training of Psychedelic Therapists,* describes best practices in the academic training of medical and mental health professionals in this field. I do highly recommend you look this up and take note of all her guidelines.

Dr. Phelps is a board member of the Heffter Research Institute, which has conducted highly influential psilocybin-assisted psychotherapy research since the 1990s. As a licensed clinical psychologist, she is a key contributor to the creation of a national accreditation board for psychedelic therapists and to methods of scaling effective training programs to meet the growing need for well-trained mental health and medical professionals in the field of psychedelic medicine.

WITNESSING AND ACKNOWLEDGING

Dr. Phelps writes from her research:

This witnessing and acknowledgment by the therapist facilitates in the participant a sense of trust, safety, encouragement, and fortitude, as is true in various modes of psychotherapy. At the same time, it solidifies the therapeutic relationship through the ebb and flow of challenges and releases during psychedelic preparation sessions and integration periods.

Phelps continues:

The therapist helps the participant move through three phases of treatment: Preparation of the medicine session, the medicine session itself, and integration of the psychological material that arises during preparation and the medicine session. The context within which this therapeutic process occurs is referred to as set and setting by Stan Grof.

Dr. Phelps referring to her colleague Stan Grof restated his definition of set and setting:

The term *set* includes the expectation, motivations, and intentions of the subject in regard to the session; the therapist's or guides concept of the nature of the LSD experience; the agreed upon goal of the psychedelic procedure; the preparation and programming of the session; and the specific techniques of guidance used during the drug experience. The term *setting* refers to the actual environment, both physical and interpersonal, and to the concrete circumstances under which the drug is administered. Dr. Phelps summarized:

In inter-subjectivity terms, these therapeutic alliances within the set and setting can be likened to the therapeutic fourth. The therapeutic fourth is the inter subjective field of set and setting that is co-created by the influence of the therapists, the psychedelic medicine, and the person ingesting the medicine.

REBIRTHING

During my training with Dr. Phelps, her key idea that she shared was:

"We are alive and watching a person birth themselves."
She views this honor and privilege as "being the witness to their birth."

Dr. Phelps described a bit of her experience working with the Peruvian Amazonian Curanderos. From them and her own experiences, she shared:

"We become the midwife to their rebirthing experience."
In doing so she suggested we need to bring the following:

- Loving kindness   • Equanimity   • Real warmth

- Compassion   • Selfless services   • Humility

- Emphatic joy

This wonderful poem originally written by Meister Eckhart reflects this eternal birthing and being fruitfully pregnant and what may come out of the process.

BIRTH

Let me express myself in even a clearer way.
The fruitful person gives birth out of the very
same foundation
from which the creator begets the eternal Word or
Creative Energy
and it is from this core
that one becomes fruitful pregnant. And in this
power of birthing
God is as fully verdant
and as wholly flourishing in full joy
and in all honoring as he/she is in him/herself.
The divine rapture
is unimaginably great.
It is ineffable.

–Meditations from Meister Eckhart by Matthew Fox
From the Teachings of Meister Eckhart

PRE-BIRTHING EXPERIENCES

Dr. Grof writes extensively about the pre-birth experiences of people being a place of exploration for healing with the non-ordinary states created by psychedelic medicine and the holotropic states. In his writings, he often refers to the birth experience as being a place where trauma may be hidden and is often overlooked. I worked with a young woman who was anorexic and bulimic and also suffered from depression and childhood sexual trauma. Although this woman had been through inpatient treatment for her eating disorder, she was unable to sustain her recovery over any long period of time. When we were in the preparation sessions meeting, before she was ready to do her KAP session, I asked her if there was anything remarkable about her birth that she remembered. She was sad to report that her mother had died the year before.

She did remember there were a lot of stories about her birth trauma and reported that her mother's uterus was half dead. While her mother was at a doctor's appointment during her pregnancy, they discovered a half-dead uterus. While my client was in the womb, her tiny heart was struggling to beat regularly and was erratic because she was literally starving in the womb. I looked at her in shock and could see what looked like a pattern and connection but it was not obvious to her.

She reported that her mother went into the hospital that day for an emergency c-section and she was born just weighing a few pounds and had to be kept in an incubator for some time. My thought was going directly to the fact that in the womb she had already been patterned for anorexia and bulimia because she would starve for a while and then eat ravenously when there were nutrients available, she gobbled the food all up. While she was in the womb there was no nutrition, and she would starve for a while to the point of having an unstable heartbeat. So, the pattern was laid into place, to a certain degree before she was born, to be anorexic and bulimic. Being in the incubator and not being held as much and soothed and comforted also played a role in some of her feelings toward her body and relationships.

During the medicine session, more of this was revealed. The client brought a blanket to the session that was a handmade quilt. She placed it over her body but did not say anything about the quilt. I kept having this thought come into my mind that was prompting me to ask her if it would be okay to wrap her in the blanket. Finally, toward the end of the medicine session, I had the strong feeling of a woman being present and asking me to wrap her in the blanket. It was already agreed upon before the session that she was okay with being touched. So, I asked her if it was okay to wrap her up in the blanket and she said yes. Then she shared that this was the last quilt that her mom made for her before her death. As I wrapped her in the blanket, with her permission, I put my arms around her as she sat on the floor and I had the feeling of her mother's arms coming right through my own arms and holding her and rocking her back and forth. We rocked for some time as she just let herself take in all the loving energy she could and feel the acceptance of herself and this new discovery of this birth pattern and how it all began. This woman left the session a different and much wiser woman. She understood her eating disorder from a much different perspective. She redid the pattern, and in her own way had a rebirth experience. And with it, the urge to binge and purge left her as well. This young woman still had some healing work to do but now she was much more empowered to live her life freer.

I always ask my clients about their birth experiences. I look deeply at the pre-birth and birth experiences and if they report any struggles to come through that birth canal and breathe that first breath of life. One woman I worked with was conceived by in vitro fertilization. She struggled with feelings like she did not belong and that she had been forced to be in the world and be in this life. I had the opportunity to ask Dr. Stan Grof at the Psychedelic Science conference in Denver, Colorado in 2023 if that would be considered a birth trauma, to be an IVF baby. He said it could have an impact.

He also commented that if they were frozen at any time, that too could have an impact with sensitivity to cold temperatures or being cold. I asked my client and she thought about it and said that she did struggle with feeling cold often and had a hard time in cold weather. This became another opportunity to look toward a rebirthing experience during her medicine session. Perhaps just looking at the IVF birth experience from a different dimension and perspective could be of help and support to others and their sense of belonging.

AN INWARD JOURNEY

Psychedelic medicine journeys, particularly with the eye shades and headphones, are typically more introverted and an inward journey. As such, the person on the journey is inwardly turned and the senses are heightened. With the psychedelic medicine journey, there can be astounding sensitivity to sights, sounds, smells, and lights. The journey can be internally rich with fractals patterns and colors. It is a place where colors can make sounds and sounds can make colors. The ancestors may come for a visit. A tree or animal may speak and share a message. A luminescent guide may communicate mind to mind without ever speaking a word.

VISITS BY WISDOM FIGURES

Within the context of the psychedelic journeys, there can be an experience of meeting wisdom figures. "I think we can meet the Master teacher," explained one friend. "We can get information, but if we don't have the grounding, we don't know what to do with the information and it can come out all distorted." So, a receptivity to knowing there may be messages and messengers on the journey, there can also be an absence of any visuals but can include an unbelievable sense of love and oneness and a feeling of being more connected to oneself and with all people and with a Power Greater than yourself.

WHAT DOES A PSYCHEDELIC EXPERIENCE FEEL LIKE?

Some people have said, "I feel really relaxed. I have a sensation of floating. I feel warmth." Or some say they are colder and need a blanket. The energy flowing in the body can feel like waves or a physical sensation, or it can feel like an electrical current pulsating a vibration that is flowing through the body.

Some people report some nausea depending on the medicine being used and some report throwing up and vomiting as part of the experience and purging. Some people report having more visuals, again depending on the psychedelic medicine.

There are many aspects that are similar or even the same on the different psychedelic journeys no matter what medicine. The difference is in the onset and how quickly the medicine comes on, the duration and the length of the journey, and the coming back and completion of the journey which are distinct or different with each type of medicine.

You're breathing and breathing exercises will help you savor the body experience and let your body do what it needs to do as your thoughts float through.

THESE EXPERIENCES HAVE BEEN REPORTED BY MANY AS PART OF THEIR PSYCHEDELIC JOURNEY:

- A lighter feeling and increased positive mood.

- Fresh thoughts about significance and meaning of objects, different life events, or seeing memories differently.

- Openness and enhanced ability to handle some distressing thoughts and memories, and the ability to see them in a more detached way.

- Ability to have less physical, mental, and emotional stress and reduced anxiety.

- Increasing of feelings of empathy or warmth and closeness to others.

- Some significant reduction in self-blame, judgment, and criticism.

- Reducing the levels of fear when looking at emotionally threatening or charged material.

- The ability to revisit personal trauma without feeling overwhelmed by the pain or shame that may have felt overwhelming in the past.

EXPLORATION ON YOUR OWN PSYCHEDELIC PATHWAYS:

What questions do you have about psychedelic medicines that still need to be answered?

....

....

....

....

What does the experience of psychedelic medicines have in potentially opening you to new realities and new dimensions of your life?

....

....

....

....

What are you most curious or concerned about with the psychedelic journey?

....

....

....

....

What type of psychedelic medicine interests you?

....

....

....

....

Do you remember your own birth story? What have you been told about your birth?

....

....

....

....

Have you experienced visits by wisdom figures, ancestors, or spiritual teachers?

....

....

....

....

3

Origin Stories

THE SECRET OF THE AGES

At the age of thirteen, my dad gave me these small magical-looking books. We called them "the red books" because they had a red leather cover with raised printing. The front cover read, "Yours is the World and Everything That's In It." There was a large hand holding the world pictured just above this phrase. Robert Collier was a clergyman and businessman from 1885 to 1950. *Secret of the Ages* was first printed in 1926, and I had been given the first edition set of six books. My grandfather was born in 1902. My father was born in 1929. When I read these books, it was 1968, and I was thirteen years old. This would be my first introduction to the meta-word, metaphysics, and the mystical transcendent realm of the Universal Mind and my Inner Healer. More of this understanding will be shared in the following section, Section Five: Spirituality and Metaphysics. Here is where it all started.

CONNECTING HEAVEN AND EARTH

Metaphysically, I learned that I could access many dimensions beyond this one. There were supernatural realms in addition to the physical worldly expression. Both realities were available and I could learn to live consciously by connecting heaven and earth—our conscious and subconscious mind. I wrote on the inside page at the age of thirteen, learning how to use the energy from the transcendent realm to be creative, solve problems, and access deeper wisdom.

CONNECTING TO MY DIVINE POWER

I read every book in the series. I underlined passages. I made a study of all the "secrets" so that I could apply them to my life. I covered the back of my bedroom door with orange-colored paper and wrote some key phrases and affirmations from the books. I read them at night before I went to sleep. I believed my dad was showing me the profound wisdom of the ages. I related to a Divine Power much greater than myself, and all the healing and transformational power of the universe was within me. I was already connected to my knowledge and healing from within. This was my first introduction to metaphysics.

MIND OUR SOURCE OF SUPPLY—NO FAILING POWERS

I underlined one of the passages, "Open up the channels between your mind and Universal Mind...There is no such thing as failing powers if we look to Mind for our source supply. The only failure of mind comes from worry and fear or from disuse. William James, the famous psychologist, taught that 'The more mind does, the more it can do.' For ideas release energy. You can do more and better work than you have ever done. You can know more than you know now. You know from your own experience that under proper mental conditions of joy and enthusiasm, you can do three or four times the work without fatigue that you can ordinarily. Tiredness is more boredom than actual physical fatigue. You can work almost indefinitely when the work is pleasurable."

ENTERING NON-ORDINARY STATES OF CONSCIOUSNESS

The path for reaching the Inner Healer and the subconscious dimensions was laid out as a three-step process in *Secret of the Ages Volume Three*. I would learn much later as I studied psychology and psychedelic medicine that the three-step process was similar for doing pre-counseling, understanding the presenting problem, taking the journey into the non-ordinary state through dreams or rituals or psychedelics, and then returning to process and do the integration work of understanding what was learned in the non-ordinary state.

The way to make contact with your subconscious mind, the way to get help of the *Inner Healer Inside You* in working out any problem is:

1. First, fill your mind with every bit of information regarding that problem that can lay your hands on.

2. Second, pick out a chair, lounge, or bed where you can recline in comfort, where you can forget your body entirely.

3. Third, let your mind dwell upon the problem for a moment,
    not worrying, not fretting, but placidly, and then turn it
    over to the Inner Healer Inside You. Say to the Inner Healer,
    this is your problem. You can do anything. You know the
    answer to what I need. Work this out for me and utterly
    relax. Drop off to sleep if you can. At least, drop into one
    of those half-sleepy, half-wakeful reveries that keep other
    thoughts from obtruding upon your consciousness.

Of course, not everyone can succeed in getting the right thought
across to the subconscious at the first or second attempt. It requires
understanding and faith, just as the working out of problems in
mathematics requires an understanding and faith in the principles
of mathematics. But keep on trying, and you will do it. And when
you do, the results are sure."

The passage went on to state, "When you awaken, hold it all
pleasurably in thought again for a few moments. Do not let doubts
and fears creep in, but go ahead, confidently, knowing your wish
is working itself out. Know this, believe it and if there is nothing
harmful in it, it will work out."

So, I began to practice this connection for many years, beginning at the age of thirteen. There was much insight gained. However,
I was also growing up and trying to find myself. I would encounter
many setbacks and testing of my newfound awareness as I went
through my teen years and into young adulthood. This metaphysical realm made a lot more sense the first time I had a psychedelic
journey and touched into the transcendent realm directly.

THE ORIGIN OF THE ORIGIN STORY

In the psychedelic community, there is a wonderful question that is often asked about your own origin story. What happened the first time you took a life-changing psychedelic journey? Or what was one of your early personal psychedelic experiences that changed you deeply in some way? Here is my origin story.

DISCLAIMER BEFORE MY ORIGIN STORY

My journey and initiation into psychedelics came at a very young age of sixteen years old. I would not recommend this for all teens. Some teens do not have the safe mindset and setting to do psychedelics and have it be a fruitful experience, and it may be overwhelming.

However, there are many unhealthy ways that teens are searching for ways to initiate themselves into adulthood, by using alcohol, recreational drug use, sex, or driving a car. Which, in America and our culture, appears to be the easiest available options. The alcohol and recreational drug use for many young people can have devastating and life-changing effects, such as: stunting emotional growth, delaying maturity into adulthood, and the possibility of addictions.

Mixing alcohol and drug use with driving a car has resulted in many young people killing themselves or someone else, and ending up in jail or prison. Sex can also be an initiation, but again, has the possibility of unintended pregnancy and is a problematic issue of children giving birth to children.

Again, without the mental, emotional, and physical means to raise a child, the weight of this is much more complicated. There is also the possibility of sexually transmitted diseases from unprotected sexual experiences.

Additionally, rape and unwanted sex, or being pushed prematurely into unwanted sexual encounters, is a massive mental, emotional, and social problem.

Historically there are cultures all around the world, which I will not go into now, that do have organized rites of passage for their young people. Some traditions involve the mindful and intentional use of the psychedelics for initiation into adulthood. In these traditions, rituals and ceremonies are done with the blessing of the tribal leaders and families. I see these as possibly useful and more mindful rites of passage into adulthood.

Personally, I did not have these tribal rituals, ceremonies, or rites of passage available to me, except through my church experience with baptism, which was powerful for me at thirteen years of age. However, by the time I reached sixteen years of age, I was ready for something more inner directed and intense. The universe provided a way for me to initiate myself with an experience of LSD. Again, I am not promoting psychedelics for teens. This is my story and my journey. Sharing this hopefully gives context to the rest of my life story and the reason I am so passionate about the mindful and intentional use of psychedelics and how I started writing about them at the age of sixteen because of one amazing English teacher.

MY ORIGIN STORY -- HAPPY 16TH BIRTHDAY!

I woke up as usual on the day of my 16th birthday. I had already experimented with a bit of marijuana, so I thought I was prepared for the experience of psychedelics. I could not have begun to understand what would happen over the next twelve hours and what I was about to enter. Before I left home for school that morning, I went into the bathroom, closed the door, and I remember looking at myself in the mirror and saying, "Happy birthday, this is going to be an interesting day!" While looking deeply into my own eyes, I took this very tiny purple microdot of acid that was given to me by a friend as my birthday gift. I remember wondering what my 16th birthday might be like. I did not know it then, but it was the day my life changed forever.

I jumped on the bus and went to school as usual. The lift off was smooth, and I went through the day much quieter and observing my classmates. It was as if I was seeing through new eyes how those around me interacted. I could read and see things from their body language so clearly that I had not paid attention to before. I was also aware that I was in a body but not limited to my body. This sounds weird, but for the first time my body felt more like a suit of clothes I was in. I was floating inside my suit of clothes that was my skin.

MIRRORS IN THE BATHROOM

I was looking for place to hang out for a bit, so I raised my hand and asked my English teacher for permission to go the bathroom. I had no experience with psychedelics and what happens when you look into mirrors. The mirrors in the girl's bathroom became my total fascination. I looked deeply in the mirror which then beautifully opened to another dimension and then another. The deeper I looked in the mirrors the more dimensions opened. I was so curious. I looked at myself and I could see that I existed on each of these multiple dimensions. I was enthralled by this vision and this new dimensional reality.

I was not the least bit afraid. I could observe different versions of myself and many portals of the universe opening at the same time. I was able to take in a vastness and connectedness that I had not directly experienced in this way. I had read of other dimensions, but I had not actually seen them or experienced them like this before. I peered more deeply into the mirror. Then bang! The big, girl's bathroom door flung open with a thud, and I was suddenly jolted back quickly from my dimensional mirror journey. I had been in the bathroom for the entire class period and my English teacher sent a girl to look for me.

My biggest mistake was telling the girl about the mirrors and what I saw and that I was tripping. She unfortunately reported this information immediately to my teacher. My teacher was very unhappy and sent me to the nurse's office. I was able to pull myself together and navigate being sent to the nurse's office to be checked out. Of course, I denied that there was anything wrong.

THE NURSE'S OFFICE

My mind was clear enough and I was able to make up a story about not feeling so well because it was "that time of the month," but I was okay now. I was just in the bathroom for a long time. The nurse was busy and quickly checked me over and released me back to class. Thankfully, she gave me a hall pass to return to my English class.

I felt a peculiar sense of openness in me and all around me as I walked back through the hallways. It was as if my mind had been closed and now was open, and there was a stream of sight and sounds that were always there, but I was hearing and seeing them for the first time. I was in an amazing heightened sensory experience. I wanted to take it all in, so I was more still, more inwardly quiet and observant. I felt as if I were suspended between two worlds, one of the expansive inner dimensions, which I could see in the mirrors that went on and on, and the other of a brick-and-mortar school building, halls, classrooms, teachers, and many noisy classrooms of students in the moment.

When I walked back into my classroom, my English teacher, Mr. Sepos, looked at me with lots of concern and suspicion. He asked, "Are you okay?" I replied that I was okay and got checked out by the nurse. Thankfully, he accepted me back into the classroom, what a big relief!

LSD BUS RIDE HOME

I went home on the bus and the bus ride gave me motion-sickness and I became nauseous. I remember throwing up a bit right after getting off the bus but feeling better. I walked home wondering how this would play out in my home with my mom, as I was still feeling the heightened effects of my LSD trip and only about six hours into what would be my twelve-hour journey.

On any normal day, I felt alone in my family and very disconnected. The psychedelics brought this reality into a sharper focus for me. I walked in the house and there was no conversation as I came in. The lack of closeness and my own despair seemed more magnified by the psychedelics. I came into my home, and I felt as though I was floating. I felt like I was an invisible ghost. I drifted in without much attention. I passed my mom and mentioned I was not feeling well, and I wanted to lie down for a bit.

She told me that I was going to go out to dinner for my birthday. I said I was not hungry and really did not want to go. She repeated with a firm frustration, "You are going out to dinner tonight," and that was it.

CARTOON CHARACTERS COMING TO LIFE

I felt a bit restless, so I went to lie down on the living room couch. My younger sister was watching cartoons. As I lie on the couch, the cartoon characters stepped out of the TV and started walking and dancing around the living room.

I found this to be amusing and it made me laugh and smile. I looked at the face of my sister and realized I was the only one who could really see this and I was enjoying it immensely. The cartoon characters walked and talked to each other, danced, and went back into the TV again. I sat there for a while feeling as though there was a universe of new experiences that I had never even thought could happen. I wondered if this visual experience was there all the time, and I just could not see it?

THE PSYCHEDELIC BIRTHDAY DINNER OUT

Although I was not the least bit hungry and did not want to go out to eat, my mother insisted we go to a terribly busy local restaurant. My mom was driving and my little sister was in the back seat. At this point my mom is noticing I am noticeably quiet, and she is inquiring what is wrong? I just kept indicating again that my stomach did not feel well but I was okay. Thank goodness she did not really push me or inquire more deeply. I was hoping she was hungry and just wanted to go out to eat. Thankfully, she believed me and stopped the questioning.

ENHANCED-SENSORY-AUDITORY STIMULATION

My hearing seemed altered and enhanced. The noise in the restaurant was too loud and intense. I could hear every conversation in detail at once. Everyone was talking at the same time about nothing at all and it all seemed so meaningless. The bright overhead lighting was overwhelming and looked like rays of rainbow crystal beams shooting randomly across the room. The lighting gave everything in the restaurant a halo effect, which illuminated everything with a glow. The dining room was pulsating in and out a bit with my heartbeat.

The colorful menu had pictures of food and as I scanned the menu, the items in the pictures kept moving around as if they were walking and animated. I was again smiling as I watched the animated food dancing on my menu. I was not able to select anything I wanted to eat so I ordered a chopped steak with mashed potatoes, which I remembered I would normally order at this restaurant every time.

DANCING CHOPPED STEAK

My dinner arrived quickly, and my chopped steak stood up on my plate. I was staring at it, chuckling silently inside. Then the chopped steak jumped off my plate. I was again smiling as I watched my chop steak do a dance and resist my trying to reach it with my fork. My mom and sister seemed oblivious and in their own worlds, eagerly eating their delicious meals. They chatted and ate but I was just sitting there smiling and trying to plan to get my chopped steak to stay on my plate. I sat quietly with fork and knife in hand. I would try to stick my fork in it, and it would move to one side. It was no use. The more I tried to get the chopped steak to stay on my plate the more it jumped and turned away from me. I did not care. I did not want to eat the chopped steak anyway. I really hated eating meat. And now as if mocking me, my chopped steak was dancing away. I stopped trying to eat it. I only wanted to watch it dance, spin, and move happily around my plate.

EATING THE FOOD THAT WAS NOT DANCING

The mashed potatoes did not move, so I decided I would eat them. The potatoes just laid in a lazy heap. They were not dancing or hopping off my plate and they became a much easier target for my fork. Soon I was eating the lumpy mashed potatoes and mom looked up and seemed satisfied. I finally asked for a to-go box, and I watched the waitress pick up my chop steak easily, as it willingly surrendered to her, and was put into a box and then bag with no problems at all. I wondered if it was still dancing in the Styrofoam container.

TWELVE HOURS LATER

I finally got home to sit in my room and just breathe and play my guitar. After about twelve hours, from 8:00 a.m. until 8:00 p.m., I was finally transported back from a place where I did not have adequate words to describe or the ability to fully comprehend. The experience was now etched in my mind so vividly, like no other memory I had ever had before. Tiny details like I am describing, I still can recall today with clarity.

PROFOUND SHIFTS IN AWARENESS
FOLLOWING MY JOURNEY

I had a psychedelic rite of passage, an initiation into something extraordinary, and I loved it. I had no fear; I was filled with curiosity and a profound sense of openness. That door of my inner world and perceptions of other dimensions had been opened. And once I opened that door, it could never be closed again.

THESE ARE THINGS I LEARNED FROM
MY VERY FIRST EXPERIENCE:

1. I was not my body—it was a suit I was wearing for a time. I had a spirit that lived in the suit that was me, but I was not the suit.

2. An expanded sense of openness and awareness of all people. I could see them more clearly and almost hear their thoughts from just being quietly aware of their presence.

3. The reality of inner and outer dimensions that are here now. That there really was no past, present, and future, and all dimensions existed at once. However, there was a choice to be present in the moment.

4. Existing on those other dimensions was more like living in a more expansive awareness of the universe. There were many dimensions beyond this one I could touch into.

5. Going beyond the normal sense of space and time. That the time I was living in was manufactured and not real; we just agreed and made it all up.

6. Sensory enhancement and vibrancy of sound, colors, and light. Everything had a vibration and energy field to it; everything was truly alive.

7. Humor and expanded sense of my creative capacity. I was deeply joyful in ways I had not experienced before. I could feel an expanded depth of my emotions and a wider array of my feelings.

MY ENGLISH TEACHER WAS MY FIRST
INTEGRATION FACILITATOR

A week after this LSD experience Mr. Sepos became my best English teacher ever. He helped me to integrate my experience with psychedelics through my writing. He helped me take my early experiences with psychedelics and turn them into something insightful through my creative writing. He said he did me a favor by not turning me in and now I needed to repay that favor by writing for the school yearbook. I agreed.

I have been a writer ever since. My writing continues to be my personal grounding, my anchor, my centering, my integration, and my internal transformational process. Mr. Sepos could have justifiably punished me and turned me in. I would have possibly been expelled from school. However, he did not do that. He used my psychedelic journey for my growth and creative development.

I do not know if he realized what he was doing. However, it turned out to be a brilliant strategy. Mr. Sepos set me in the direction of my future path. He was my first psychedelic integration facilitator. He would never know that one day, many years later, I would become a psychotherapist, a commercially published author on self-help, healing, and personal transformation, and work in Psychedelic-Assisted Psychotherapy. Instead of putting me down, he lifted me up, and Mr. Sepos made me use my psychedelic experiences for good. He challenged me to write about my inner-world experiences. Some of my thoughts reflected in this poem I wrote at age sixteen for our yearbook, following my LSD journey:

THE DOORS I OPEN

The rest of my life will be involved
in personal experiences and on-the-job-training.
The decisions I make will be the ones I will have to live with;
The doors I open can be closed only by me.
I pray for the strength to stand up for all
I believe:
I pray for fortitude to bear all the failure I must encounter.
I pray for help to smooth out the bumps in life's path.
I pray for my friends.

DOORS OF PERCEPTIONS

Years later, reading Aldous Huxley's *Doors of Perception,* it reminded me of this place I had entered within myself. I had opened the doors of my "inner perception," as Huxley would say. I was now experiencing my own kaleidoscope of thoughts and feelings. The textures of these inner worlds encouraged me to look beyond the one-dimensional world and look inwardly with my interior eyes and ears and senses turned toward the inner dimensions, the secrets within.

Huxley points to an interesting urge that we all have, "The urge to transcend self-conscious selfhood is... a principal appetite of the soul." I felt this urge early in my teen years. I have continued to peruse and feed my soul life consistently, in as healthy ways as possible, through a variety of pathways of dreams, rituals, and psychedelics.

WHAT IS YOUR ORIGIN STORY?

Do you have an origin story? Capture a few thoughts.

....

....

....

....

What did your first experience teach you, or how did it change your view of your life?

....

....

....

....

How were you changed, if at all, following the experience?

....

....

....

....

What perceptions shifted or changed for you?

....

....

....

....

Triune
Pathway Two:
Dreams

Chapter Four describes how dreams are a boundless pathway to non-ordinary states of consciousness and how to combine them with psychedelics and rituals. We enter this dream realm nightly. We are flying, talking to people who have passed on, and doing time travel to different dimensions and places in this world and beyond.

Chapter Five gives a brief yet insightful look at metaphysics and mysticism. We can better understand consciousness through psychedelics, and an understanding of metaphysics can help with integration. There is a paradigm shift taking place where we become our own inner healers and our own seers and allow a space for our own inner truths to be revealed directly. In the mystical experience, revelations can and do happen during non-ordinary states of consciousness.

Chapter Six addresses Ego Death, one of the top anxiety-provoking fears: the fear of dying. Everyone will one day make the transition from this life and leave their physical body behind. In this chapter, we explore how to face our dying more consciously and how psychedelics and dreams can play an important role in transcending the fears around death and perhaps help to answer some of the existential questions of life and the end of life.

4

Dreams and Inner Transformation

WHAT YOUR DREAMS ARE SAYING TO YOU?

We dream every night. Dream images are transmissions. They are always there waiting for us to tune in to them. No one can really tell you what your dreams mean to you, but you. Dream imagery is highly individualistic and personal, only you can provide the context for your dream's meaning. They are your inner messaging system to yourself, often cryptic in their symbol and rich in their archetypal dimensions.

Dreams have always been a way for me to receive guidance, to enter the non-ordinary states. I write them down every night, and they have a big impact on my life. Dreams are one of the most powerful pathways to enter our existential human experience and help us on some level, answer the questions: What is the meaning of my life? What is the purpose of my life?

I have kept a dream journal for over thirty years now. These dream messengers provide my guidance for many things that have come up in my life and relationships. Dreams are ways to help us contact a Higher Wisdom, our Inner Healer, our Higher Self.

A RECORD OF YOU BECOMING

One woman who keeps a journal shared,

> "The journal, and my dreams in it, record the secret part of my life. In doing that, my journal makes me whole to myself. It is my ever-changing blueprint of the piece of work that I become. Only together with my journal and dreams do I make it possible to produce a product, called my life experience. And the combination of my journal and my dreams does not present all I am, it records my becoming. Then I live that out, one day at a time, and I know where and what I am in that way."

We can ask for a dream to help us understand what is happening in our life. When we are disturbed, we can write in our journal about our feelings and get in the flow of our inner guidance and movement of our life. We can feel ourselves as channels through which wisdom flows to bring the guidance we need. Find someone that you can share your dreams with. As you hear yourself sharing your dreams, you will gain new insights. Decide that you are going to listen to your dreams, that you are willing to change, you are willing to grow. You are willing to give consent to the higher action with you. Willingness always proceeds growth and change.

Sometimes, our Higher Self, our Inner Healer, is trying to teach us something, and the human mind or ego blocks it. The dreams might come, and we are unable to relate them to our life experiences. Write it down, and later, when you are ready to work, you can go back to read your dreams and you will be able to listen to what it is trying to say to you. The light will dawn! We need to give permission to ourselves to move out of the negative, boxed-in attitudes and be free to do what needs to be done by us.

WORKING WITH UNDERSTANDING YOUR DREAMS

1. Believe that dreams are of value.

2. Invite your dreams before you sleep, using a thought such as: I am open to guidance from my dreams tonight.

3. Keep a journal and pen next to the bed or some way to record your dreams. Voice memos on your phone could work as well. Record all you can remember of your dream in the night or immediately upon waking in the morning. Also write down what is going on with your life currently. Be sure to date your dream record.

4. Meditate on your dream or the feeling you have in the morning. You can ask, "Help me understand this dream or feeling I have." Then be quiet and receptive. It is good to again write down what comes.

5. Keep a journal and write down other experiences in your inner life: images, songs, ideas, coincidences, promptings, the way things work out, remembrances, intimations of things coming, intuitive sensing, or life situations that you feel are trying to tell you something.

6. Befriend your dreams. Have love and patience toward them and what they must tell you. Be positive toward them.

7. Relate to your dreams. Ask questions of the dream or people or things in the dream, such as, "What are you to me or in my life?" And then enter the silence and listen. You may to discuss your dream with an aware person.

Have a sense of gratitude for the dreams, your deep wisdom for the many ways this dream speaks to you and strengthens you. You are here to live and demonstrate wonderful happenings because there is a great wisdom, a great love, a great peace, a great power living through you.

DIFFERENT TYPES OF DREAMS

Nightmares: Often occur during times of stress and trying to get the conscious and unconscious mind to work together. There may be factors influencing the nightmare, particularly internal psychological factors, and stressful external life changes.

Lucid Dreams: In these dreams you are awake and know you are awake while you are dreaming and can have more influence on the way the dream plays out.

Problem-Solving Dreams: In these dreams there is a new perspective revealed or some solution to a problem. Many inventions, including the sewing machine, have come from these types of dreams.

Symbolic Dreams: Metaphorically, something is revealed which gives some insight or instruction. The symbol can be viewed as a part of our self-knowing personal development and insight.

Telepathic Dreams: There are messages given in the dream that reveal something that has happened in another place that you may or may not know has happened, but the dream realm has the extrasensory ability to perceive it.

Pleasure Dreams: These dreams can be like mini vacations during the night or serve to give some comfort to someone with something. The fantasy is lived out in the dream and can reduce anxiety and bring some needed internal self-soothing.

Communal or Mutual Dreams: This is a shared dream experience where you and others share the same or similar dreams at the same or similar time.

Current Event Dreams: Things going on in your life, your community, your workplace, your country, or the world may come up within dreams. These representations may be metaphoric or symbolic as well.

Visitation Dreams: These are dreams characterized by a visit from an ancestor or a person who has recently died. A family member, pet, or friend may come to visit in your dreams. These dreams may also include Divine Beings, wisdom teachers, and historical figures.

Spiritual Dreams: These dreams are often revelations, sometimes prophetic, and can show something beyond this world in the spiritual or transpersonal dimensions of life.

Premonition Dreams. The future is being revealed in some way and can show a vision of what is going to be. In this dream, a future event may be shown that comes true later.

Healing Dreams: These dreams often show or point to something that is important for the healing of the mind, body, or spirit.

Recurring Dream: These dreams repeat themselves over and over with the same scene playing repeatedly.

One good way to find answers to your dream questions is through the dialogue process. You can dialogue with the characters of images in the dreams and let them speak to you and open the messages enveloped in your dream. By dialoguing, and talking to the parts of your dream, you learn to hear the things that will open your ears to inner resources.

MEDITATION BEFORE SLEEP TO INVITE DREAMS

Some say they never dream. But the fact is we all dream every night, we just might not remember our dreams. Reading this brief meditation before bedtime can be an invitation to your dreams welcoming them to come. Be sure to have a way to record them on your phone or in a written journal. Even a few lines or words can be a tiny thread you pull to bring back the whole dream.

Here is the meditation to read before going to sleep:

I dream the dreams of my inner healing intelligence. My dreams tonight will draw me closer to my right fulfillment. My dreams are healing influences. They are messengers to me creating, unifying, restoring, and renewing me. My dreams expand my consciousness into the cosmic consciousness so that I am more aware of the treasures of life and have good success in the projects I am guided to undertake. My dreams bring me into a whole new relationship with my environment. My involvement with society is made more responsible and interesting. Negative thought patterns, old scripts, or stories about myself are revealed and constructively changed through revelations in my dreams tonight. All fears, inferiority feelings, hatreds, and guilts which are destructive, are shown to me clearly, as undesirable. I am shown my spiritual power and my deepest self-compassion which transforms my whole soul into a healthier me. My dreams express my fuller potential and invigorate my life with infinite energy. If it is important for me to remember a dream, I will remember it. My dreams affect my thinking, feeling, speech, and behavior patterns as I meditate and go about the everyday business of my life. I am much more intuitive, emphatic, and highly aware. I know the things I need to know easily. Good flows to me from every direction and I am grateful.

WORKING THE FOUR STEP APPROACH
TO WORKING WITH DREAMS

One of my favorite teachers that I had the chance to study with was Robert Johnson, the Jungian Analyst, who was the author of the books *He* and *She*, another one of my favorites *Ecstasy*, and for doing personal dream work, *Inner Work: Using Dreams and Active Imagination for Personal Growth*. Here is what I have found to be an easy and effective way to work with my dreams.

Robert Johnson has a basic four step method for approaching our dreams:

1. Making associations.

2. Connecting dream images to inner dynamics.

3. Interpreting.

4. Doing rituals to make the dream concrete.

Johnson goes on to explain:

> In the first step, we form the foundation for interrupting the dream by finding the association that spring out of our unconscious in response to the dream images. Every dream is made up of a series of images, so our work begins with discovering the meanings that those images have. In the second step, we look for and find the parts of our inner selves that the dream images represent. We find the dynamics at work inside us that are symbolized by the dream situation. Then, in the third step, the interpretation, we put together the information we have gleaned in the

first two steps and arrive at a view of the dream's meaning when taken as a whole. In the fourth step, we learn to do rituals that will make the dream more conscious, imprint its meaning more clearly on our minds, and give it the concreteness of immediate physical experience.

Johnson views ritual and ceremony as a valuable pathway to reconnect us with the unconscious realms. For some people, this may be a challenging step of the dream work. Johnson reflects, "When I ask, what are you going to *do* about your dream? they draw a blank. Yet, with a little practice, you learn to use your imagination and invent ingenious rituals that will give your dream immediacy and physical concreteness. You will be surprised at how much power this fourth step has to intensify your understanding of the dream, and even to change your habits and attitudes." These ritual acts can be concrete actions or symbolic actions. Any small action will do.

PAUL STAMETS DREAM AND MUSHROOM EXPERINCES

Historically, and for thousands of years, plant-based medicines were used by shamans and healers as earth-based natural medicines, and to protect their communities from dangers and disasters. Paul Stamets, author and world-renowned mycologist, reflects on this intersection between the psychedelic journey and the world of dreams in this recounting of a story from his life experience. A friend of Paul's had discovered a large patch of naturally-grown psychedelic mushrooms growing in a patch directly across from a Seattle police station. Paul and his friends went and picked and harvested the mushrooms and made some of them into psychedelic smoothies.

Paul Stamets shared about the psychedelic experience after drinking the smoothie:

> In twenty minutes, we started to experience the first stages of lift off. The first hour is often the most unsettling part of the experience; later stages bring a familiar reassurance. Two hours into the experience, we could sense a slowing of intensity, and at three hours we plateaued. The dose was strong and richly rewarding. Unfolding geometric patterns surged towards me in wave after wave of beauty and complexity. My thoughts centered on God, evolution, the living earth, the infinite universe, the forces of good and evil, the mystery of death, and the paradox of time.

PAUL'S DREAM JOURNEY

Following the journey, Paul had dozed off to sleep and was visited by a foreshadowing dream. Paul reported,

> An hour or two past midnight, about six hours from the first mushroom smoothie, I went to bed. Geometric patterns continued to light up my field of vision as I descended into sleep. Several hours later, in a twilight between sleep and wakefulness, a peculiar and strangely real dream enveloped me. I was in college, desperately trying to return to my mountain cabin as if my life depended upon it. This sense of urgency preempted all other priorities. Go back. Go back quickly. In dream state, I drove hurriedly into the mountains. Then turning a corner on a country road, I came into a broad river valley lit up with a cold,

clear light. The valley had flooded. Floating, dead, and bloated in the frigid sunlight were hundreds and hundreds of cows. The dream abruptly ended, and I awoke in a cold sweat, struck with a fear of impending disaster.

PAUL'S DOOMSDAY

Paul was compelled to share his dream with his friends. He goes on to say:

This was like no dream I had ever had; there was a particularly foreboding strangeness to it that struck to the very core of my being. I feared there would be something like a nuclear war...the USSR would attack, the snow would melt from the heat of the nuclear fireballs, and cows would be killed from the ensuing floods! My friends, not taking me seriously, began to joke. However, one person was curious enough to ask when this catastrophe would strike. I told him it would happen soon...I did not know when, except that I knew it would be on a weekend. He pointed to a date on the calendar two weeks out, December 1, and I knew that was it. He wrote, 'Paul says Doomsday' on that date, and the conversation changed course.

Paul astonishingly describes what happened two weeks later:

Two weeks later, after torrential rains and nearly record-breaking snowfall in the Cascades, and unusual temperature inversion swept over western Washington. Temperatures soared in the mountains, and the sudden thaw turned brooks into raging rivers in a matter of hours. Trees, houses, and bridges were flooded. My cabin, located only twenty feet from a glacial creek, was in immediate jeopardy. I knew that if I could not return quickly, all could be lost-my reference books, my manuscripts, all my personal belongings. The next day, I drove back to Darington only to meet closures at one bridge after another. Finally, I drove a circuitous route, adding a hundred miles to my trek, to find that my cabin was still safe but now ten feet closer to the raging river. The next day, I packed everything and headed out to Olympia. As I entered the Snohomish Valley, I stared in disbelief at hundreds of cattle who, standing by the rising waters, had drowned overnight. It was December 1, the exact day my dream had foretold. This single event shattered my concept of linear time. The future can be foreseen. Now I knew what shamans have known for centuries: the psilocybin experience can facilitate precognition of the future-especially, as in my case, of an impending biological disaster. Now I understand why the Mazatec and Aztecs affectionately referred to Psilocybes as divinatory mushrooms, genius mushrooms, and wondrous mushrooms. They recognized that mushrooms are powerful sacraments and a significant evolutionary advantage for those sensitive enough to heed the call.

THE MUSHROOM IS YOUR TEACHER

Paul has been a trailblazer, far ahead of the pack, and has led the way to bring these sacred mushrooms back into our lives. He concludes by suggesting, "The path is ancient, noble, and for many, holy. I hope that you will discover the capacity of the mushrooms to lead to a new type of consciousness. Be careful, observant, respectful, and wise. The mushroom will be your teacher."

Personally, meeting my teacher, Paul Stamets, at the International Conference on Psychedelic Research in the Netherlands, was a highlight of my life. Of course, I highly recommended his book, *Psilocybin Mushrooms of the World,* to guide you on your journey as Paul has helped guide me on mine.

Today plant-based medicines and psychedelic mushrooms are once again valued as new tools available for inner healing. There is a new resurgence and education on how mushrooms can be used in psychotherapy. For the first time in recent history, we have new tools in the proverbial toolbox. Our new medicine bag includes MDMA, synthetic psilocybin, ketamine, and more. There is a receptivity and openness for plant medicines, and integration work with healing experiences of non-ordinary states.

QUESTIONS FOR DREAM UNDERSTANDING:

What types of dreams have you had that stand out for you?

....

....

....

....

What important messages have you received in your dreams?

....

....

....

....

What life-changing dreams have influenced or guided you?

....

....

....

....

Have you ever been warned or shown something to be aware of in your dreams?

....

....

....

....

5

Metaphysics and Mysticism

KNOWING BEYOND KNOWING

It is the closing of our outer eyes and looking within with our inner eyes. Sometimes we can see so much more when our eyes are closed, and we go within. As we do, we may touch into an energetic field of universal awareness. Sometimes referred to as "knowing beyond knowing" as a way that looks past the physical outer world and peers into the heart of ourselves and our own beliefs and metaphysical underpinnings. Entering the inner space of all potentialities. Touching the golden thread of our highest Self, our best Self, our higher energy, our inner healer.

MEDICINE IS THE CATALYST

Psychedelic medicine opens the pathway. The medicine is a catalyst for this experience. There are many pathways through meditation, dreaming, breathwork, ritual and ceremony, drumming, chanting, and walking a labyrinth are all ways we may touch into the mystical realms. Once we have these spiritual connections and experiences, they need to be woven into our daily lives and made practical, usable, and sustainable for the whole self to benefit.

We are learning how to bring this into our daily thoughts, making the unseen seen, the invisible visible, and entering the darkness to see the light. The inner work to maintain the connection to the spiritual realm is through mindfulness. To bring forth our best self, our truest self, is the journey to love, wisdom, and power. We are actualizing more of ourselves consciously to enter more fully the place of our own personal enlightenment and transformation. This does not just randomly happen; this inner work is intentional, and that is why we set our intentions before the journey.

We are intentionally doing our inner work. Conversely, psychedelic medicine, done simply for recreational intentions, may bring out things that are unintegrated. Not processed with a skilled therapist or facilitator, it may not be maintained or captured to have the fullest potential for life transformation and healing. There is an experience, but without the insight of what it means to your life. Like a dream, it is a weird visual experience, and looking at it from a more interpretative standpoint enlivens and informs our lives. Inviting a qualified therapist or facilitator is an important collaborative piece.

WHAT ARE METAPHYSICS AND MYSTICISM?

The path of metaphysics, mysticism, and psychedelics are intersections that are essential to understanding and gaining perspective on the inner world and the psychedelic pathway. Each of these is needed to truly know the other. Let's start with some basic definitions.

WHAT IS METAPHYSICS?

Metaphysics is the branch of philosophy that deals with the first principles of things, including abstract concepts, such as being, knowing, substance, cause, identity, time, and space. Metaphysics is a type of study that uses broad concepts to help define reality and gain some understanding of it. Metaphysical studies seek to explain inherent or universal elements of reality that are not easily discovered or experienced in our everyday ordinary waking consciousness. This is why it is important to take time to enter non-ordinary states of consciousness where we can touch into this pathway.

Derived from the Greek meta ta physika ("after the things of nature"); referring to an idea, doctrine, or situated reality *outside* of human sense perception. In philosophical terminology, metaphysics refers to the study of what cannot be reached through objective studies of material reality.

THERE ARE A FEW TOPICS OF
METAPHYSICAL INVESTIGATION:

- Existence.

- Cause and effect.

- Objects and their properties.

- Possibility.

- Space and time.

METAPHYSICS IS THE BRANCH OF PHILOSOPHY THAT EXAMINES THE FUNDAMENTAL NATURE OF REALITY, INCLUDING:

- The relationship between mind and matter.

- Between potentiality and actuality.

- Between substance and attribute.

In the book, *Practical Metaphysics: A New Insight in Truth*, author Eric Butterworth says, that metaphysics literally means "beyond the science of nature."

Academically, metaphysics is the branch of philosophy that studies the ultimate reality beyond the physical realm and generally asks these questions:

- What is the nature of being?

- How do we know what we know?

- What is the nature of the universe?

Some meta-physicians like Butterworth may also ask:

- What is the nature of the Inner Healer/God and humankind?

- What is the relationship between the Inner Healer/God and humankind?

The Inner Healer is the invisible life and intelligence underlying all physical things. And as the inner healing intelligence underlies all things, our Inner Healer can also be referred to as Divine Mind, Universal Mind, and Cosmic Consciousness. According to the book *The Revealing Word*, by Charles Fillmore, metaphysics is defined as "The systematic study of the science of Being: that which transcends the physical." Think about that for a minute, the science of Being. What is the intelligence underlying all things? That is what metaphysics is looking at.

Metaphysics would look at the perception or revelation of the "unseen" as being as real as the "seen." Metaphysics is the place where the *unseen is real.*

Eric Butterworth goes on to describe how this manifest in our lives by suggesting, "The personality/ego must surrender to the divine essence within and then awaken to its wisdom. That surrender is what allows the demonstration to flow through us." He goes on to state, "We do not 'demonstrate' so much as we allow the 'imprisoned splendor' to escape." So, it takes a surrender of what we have come to know as reality, and surrendering to a greater reality that is connected to something we don't often touch in our daily waking consciousness. So, in this sense, we are all prophets, seers, sages, and saviors in the making, as we are releasing our own imprisoned splendor and letting our light shine and therefore bringing the kingdom of light and oneness to illuminate our world and the world around us.

What this means is that we can have direct knowledge of the Divine right now. We have direct access to the awakening of the wisdom within us. When places of worship are truly safe and welcoming, religious institutions play an important role as centers where people can join in the community and develop supportive relationships with others. Religious institutions and their religious leaderships are not a prerequisite to having a spiritual experience or firsthand wisdom and a direct experience of the Divine. Religious institutions do play an important social gathering role in our communal life. There is immense value in having a place to gather, celebrate rites of passage, serve one another, and help uplift and heal communities of people. Many people in different world religions continue to orient themselves in the world through their spiritual practices in churches, synagogues, temples, and mosques.

The new paradigm, which is in truth, thousands of years old, just more hidden, is the direct knowledge of the Divine, or Gnosis. Gnosis is an immanent form of knowledge or transcendent insight, and it is the process of knowing. The word Gnosis is a Greek word that means knowledge. It comes from an Indo-European root gno, from which the English word "knowledge" comes. In the time of the Late Antiquity, the word Gnosis was used to designate an intuitive awareness of hidden mysteries as opposed to analytical knowledge that was derived from classes, books, or liturgies and lectures from others.

OPENING TO YOUR INNER SPLENDOR

Yielding and allowing the imprisoned splendor to flow through us is part of the psychedelic journey. This yielding allows us to enter a more metaphysical understanding of what lies beyond the physical realm and supports us all the time. There is an innermost truth and healing that exists constantly. It is more of a perception than anything outer, it is an inner shifting. It allows the light within to glow brilliantly. This beautiful poem by Robert

Browning describes this "truth" that is within us all the time. It is a clarity of perception that is available within our own being.

Paracelsus

Truth is within ourselves; it takes no rise
From outward things, whate'er you may believe.
There is an inmost center in us all,
Where truth abides in fullness; and around,
Wall upon wall, the gross flesh hems it in,
This perfect, clear perception--which is truth.
A baffling and perverting carnal mesh
Binds it, and makes all error; and to know
Rather consists in opening out a way
Whence the imprisoned splendor may escape,
Than in effecting entry for a light
Supposed to be without.

WHAT IS MYSTICISM

Very simply, it is the experience of the mystical union or direct communion with ultimate reality reported by mystics. It is a belief that the direct knowledge of God, spiritual truth, or ultimate reality, can be attained through subjective experience, for example, intuition or insight.

Mysticism can be any kind of ecstasy or non-ordinary state of consciousness which is given spiritual meaning. It may be described as the experience of becoming one with God or the Absolute. There may be capabilities of knowing beyond knowing, seeing beyond seeing, hearing, and attaining knowledge or information from an extraordinary access to a source beyond and possessing the power to have dominion with this knowledge in more meaningful ways. It may include finding a place of sanctuary in the transcendent realm of the supernatural world. The belief that union with or absorption in the Deity or absolute, or the spiritual understanding of knowledge inaccessible to the intellect, may be attained through contemplation and self-surrender. Here is why understanding both metaphysics and mysticism can help with dreams, rituals, and psychedelics.

IMPORTANT TO UNDERSTAND THE FOLLOWING ABOUT METAPHYSICS AND MYSTICISM:

1. We can have a mystical experience and not understand metaphysics. A flash of light, the appearance of a deity, and a revelation can happen to anyone. If we have some sense of metaphysics and a larger understanding to see the experience from the mystical experience, we will have a better place to take root and inform our inner and outer lives.

2. The metaphysical underpinnings simply help us to understand there is a dimension beyond time and space where these mystical experiences can and do emerge with their *splendor* being revealed. Beyond the ego-encapsulated flesh, there is a light and splendor we can touch when we take a medicine journey.

3. From a metaphysical dimension, we can be our own seer and have a direct revelation of a mystical nature. We are our own sages and can have a direct experience of knowing. By entering the mystical union, we can understand ourselves and the ineffable more deeply. We can receive these revelations in our own mystical union.

4. Without some understanding of the intersection of metaphysics, mysticism, and psychedelics, there may be a loss of integration for the fullest meaning of our experiences. People may have some revelations, but they need to be understood, and what is revealed is applicable to healing and transforming the whole person.

For example, I had a dream visitation experience one night of Jesus appearing at the foot of my bed. For me, it was a direct experience or revelation of the numinous, opening me to the Spirit. This was one of the deepest experiences I have ever had of oceanic oneness. The confidence of the visit conveyed a presence and that I was not alone. Jesus was with me, and I was being guided in ways I could not begin to understand. The touching of the ineffable was like touching the hem of Jesus's garment and having the visceral response and energy flow directly through me. I was healed of the fears holding me back.

It was a true visitation for me, a revelation and mystical vision in my dream. These experiences are possible to have without using any psychedelic medicines. These mystical experiences can and often do happen spontaneously, particularly in our dream state. So, the non-ordinary state can be entered, and knowledge revealed as a mystical experience directly with revelations with or without psychedelics.

KNOWLEDGE OF THE SACRED

One incredible therapist trained in theology and the psychology of religion with decades of experience working with people and helping them enter non-ordinary states of consciousness with psychedelics is Dr. Bill Richards. A psychologist in the Psychiatry Department of the Johns Hopkins University School of Medicine, Bayview Medical Center, a consultant, and trainer at sites of psychedelic research internationally, a teacher in the Program of Psychedelic-Therapy and Research at the California Institute of Integral Studies (CIIS). I met Bill in the Netherlands in 2022 and experienced a full-day workshop with him and Dr. Janis Phelps, the Director of the CIIS program, which trains psychedelic therapists. The only sanctioned educational institution at the time, training psychedelic therapists. They were joined by Dr. Torsten Passie, a psychiatrist and psychotherapist, working for decades with psychedelic medicines.

Dr. Richards, who likes to be called Bill, wrote the book, *Sacred Knowledge: Psychedelics and Religious Experiences*, which I highly enjoyed and recommend. Reflecting on the mystical consciousness he writes, "The core of this book is about the nature and relevance of mystical consciousness, and the visionary experiences that sometimes precede, or follow, or accompany this unspeakably vast, dynamic, magnificent, and profoundly meaningful state of awareness."

NAMING ULTIMATE REALITY

Richards goes on to share that this is something at the deep recesses of all our beings that we are already connected to. He suggested that it goes by many names of those who have had their kind of inner death and rebirth experiences. Some of the names are "Cosmic Consciousness" or "Ultimate Reality." Richards goes on to state, "All of the great world religions have words that point toward this highly desired and valued state of spiritual awareness, such as *samadhi* in Hinduism, *nirvana* in Buddhism, *sekhel mufla* in Judaism, *the beatific vision* in Christianity, *baqa' wa fana'* in Islam, and *wu wei* in Taoism."

Dr. Richards goes on to say, "Although there may be room for infinite variations in the nature and descriptions of individual reports of these experiences, which have delighted scholars of mystical literature and researchers of meditative states of consciousness in years past and will continue to occupy them long into the future, the research with psychedelic substances surveyed strongly supports the reality of a common core of characteristics and the validity of what Robert K.C. Forman has called the 'Pure Consciousness Event' or PCE."

PURE CONSCIOUSNESS EVENT: PCE

The "common core" reliability includes descriptions of:

1. Unity.
2. Transcendence of Time and Space.
3. Intuitive Knowledge.
4. Sacredness.
5. Deeply Felt Positive Mood.
6. Ineffability.

UNIVERSAL KEYS THAT UNLOCK THE DOOR

After decades of observing volunteer patients go through the research with psychedelics, which he likes to call entheogens, Dr. Richards has concluded, "It is reasonable to view these psychedelics substances as different skeleton or universal keys that can unlock the door within each of our minds to other forms of consciousness, essentially providing an opportunity for exploration and discovery rather than a particular discrete form of experiences."

So, in essence, each substance may have its own speed of action and produce a variety of results. Each experience is one of a kind for that individual on that day and will never be repeated in the same way again, even with the same substance. Dr. Richards states, "In my experience, the range of alternative states of consciousness facilitated by LSD, DPT, psilocybin, and DMT, is very similar, if not identical.

THE SUBSTANCES PRIMARILY APPEAR TO DIFFER FROM ONE ANOTHER IN TERMS OF:

- Speed of onset.
- Arc and length of action.
- And abruptness of returning one to the everyday world.

UNDERSTANDING CONSCIOUSNESS THROUGH PSYCHEDELICS

Dr. Peter Sjostedt-Hughes, professor of philosophy and metaphysics suggested to me at a recent workshop sponsored by the International Conference on Psychedelic Research (ICPR) in 2022, that all psychotherapists working with psychedelics needed a basic understanding of metaphysics. I said that I agreed. Peter asked me if I thought they would be open and willing to learn more. I said yes and that I was writing about it and hoped this would help.

Dr. Sjostedt-Hughes pointed out how much of our idea of consciousness was gathered from Plato, and that Plato had been immersed in the Eleusinian Mysteries. The Eleusinian Mysteries were initiations held every year for the followers of Demeter and Persephone based at the Panhellenic Sanctuary of Elefsina in ancient Greece. The initiations are some of the most famous of the secret religious rites held in ancient Greece. Some scholars believe that the fungi ergot, containing LSD-like psychedelic alkaloids, were ingested as part of the ceremony, functioning as an entheogen. Plato reported that he fasted and then drank a prescribed potion and then wrote the following after having one of his own psychedelic experiences, "We saw the blessed sight and vision and were initiated into that which is rightly called the most blessed mysteries." He also wrote, "We looked upon perfect apparitions, which we saw in the pure light, being ourselves pure and not entombed in this which we carry about with us call the body, in which we are imprisoned like an oyster in its shell." -Plato (Phaedrus, 250b-c)

Dr. Sjostedt-Hughes described how through psychedelics we can explore what consciousness is and can be. He suggested, through just one experience there can be a deeper appreciation for all of nature a sense that all organisms have sentience and conscious awareness. There can be a firsthand experience of the alterations of time and space, and at the same instant, a moving beyond self-consciousness and having a knowing of being a part of an entire realm of consciousness that goes far beyond our everyday thoughts and beliefs. He states, "Psychedelics should once more be taken seriously as intellectual and aesthetic instruments that can help us understand what consciousness is but what we humans really are and what we can become in relation to the wonder that is nature."

WE ARE SPIRITUAL BEINGS HAVING HUMAN
EXPERIENCES: PIERRE TEILHARD DE CHARDIN

Teilhard recognized this spiritual beingness in all of us as our primary state of being. From my own perspective and experience, we talk a great deal about the healing of mind, body, and spirit, but tend to leave out our spirit. Our spirit is innately a part of our inner world. It is a part already present and naturally occurring. Knowing we are spiritual beings having a human experience helps us understand our journey of life from a fresh perspective. We are not human beings trying to become more spiritual, we are innately spiritual beings having human experiences. The spiritual awareness will hopefully help us to learn and grow through these experiences. Understanding some basics of spirituality and metaphysics helps us have a broader framework beyond the therapeutic neuroscience realm for the psychedelic experience to be viewed and understood from another perspective. This is a very simplified version of a much more complicated and deeply intellectual view that has its underpinnings in the great philosophers of our time.

So, we have a body, but we are not our bodies. It is simply a vehicle to transport our beingness and consciousness around in our daily life experiences. We have thoughts but we are not our thoughts. We have many and varied feelings, but we are not our feelings. Thoughts and feelings are something that we experience following a sensory experience. Each person will have their own unique thoughts and feelings following each sensory life experience. The same thing could happen to two different people, but they have a variety of different thoughts and feelings about it.

When I am working with a person in counseling and doing psychedelic-assisted therapy, I do not announce, "I am going to be working with you spiritually, metaphysically, or mystically now." I hold the intention of this in my heart and mind even before I meet with the person. This might be more akin to how the shamans and medicine people might work; they know they are already connected to the Great Spirit. It is already happening for us all at some level; we are already connected to the allness and oneness in our spiritual dimension and knowing.

DROP OF DIVINITY

We begin to understand from a spiritual, metaphysical sense that we come from the "allness and the oneness." We might say we are like a drop of the ocean, appearing to be a separate drop, but not knowing we are always and forever a part of the ocean. The Divine Spirit is the metaphoric ocean. Beginning to connect with the ocean brings us to the awareness of being part of something much larger and greater than ourselves. There is a Power Greater than ourselves and we are swimming in it all the time. We are not the power, as our ego wants to sometimes think. We are a part of the Power and the Divine, just as the drop is part of the ocean.

We begin to understand and consciously connect with the Power Greater than ourselves. We listen to the calling from our Inner Healer, our inner healing consciousness, or whatever name feels right for us. This awareness may or may not be something the person I am working with is consciously aware of. At some point, this becomes clear that this is going on all the time whether they are consciously aware of it or not. Being conscious of this presence and Power can greatly facilitate the therapeutic potential. My favorite affirmation I wrote for myself and shared with hundreds of clients over the years is: *"I alone must do it, but I never do it alone."* Please use this affirmation daily to stay aware of the energetic connection we all have to a Power Greater than ourselves all the time.

GOING BEYOND MY PERSONAL LIFE TRAUMAS

On my personal journeys with psychedelic medicine, I noticed there was a looking back into the jar of my trauma. The psychedelics shared an even bigger view, a larger mental image or picture, so I could see the whole jar and all around it from a different perspective. There was an expansive and mystical component. More was shown to me and clearly revealed during my psychedelic medicine journey. As a result, I could have more self-compassion.

Accompanying this revelation was a deep connectedness at the core of my being with a loving and healing presence. For me, this is always a part of the light that appears, and often my Divine Mother's presence. I touched the sacredness of my own life through a mystical loving connection with something so much greater than myself, and it healed me from the inside and then radiated outwardly and touched every aspect of my life and relationships. For me, it was a mystical therapeutic transcendence.

I worked with a man who had a history of trauma both from his work as a police officer and from a dysfunctional marriage he had stayed in for many years. Tears of joy and ecstasy flowed when the Divine Mother Mary came to him and wrapped him in a warm blue shimmer light. He felt her arms totally wrap around him as she gently rocked him in her arms and took away all the hurt and suffering. It was as though she could absorb it all into herself and he surrendered to the healing balm she generously offered him. Mary gave him a message that was for me as well.

The Mystical Connections (MEQ) are very similar to the Pure Consciousness Event (PCE) in their findings.

MYSTICAL CONNECTIONS

The original Mystical Experience Questionnaire (MEQ) was a thirty-question exploration designed by Walter Pahnke to explore some of the nuances of the mystical experience with psychedelics.

THERE WERE FOUR AREAS THAT
WERE INITIALLY EXPLORED:

1. Factor One: Mystical

2. Factor Two: Positive Mood

3. Factor Three: Transcendence of Time and Space

4. Factor Four: Ineffability

MY OWN MYSTICAL FACTORS: APPEARANCE
OF THE DIVINE MOTHER

During a psychedelic medicine session, the Divine Mother appeared to me. I felt as though I was being fed the light of her Spirit going directly into me. My only way to describe this was that it was like being fed the mother's milk emanating from her own heart which was nourishing and feeding me at the deepest soul and cellular level of my being.

Metaphysically, for me, this was my Spiritual Mother coming to me from another dimension of time and space to nourish and feed me with her divine splendor, her light, which gave me strength and healing in every dimension of my own being. My sense of separateness dropped away. I was one with my Spiritual Mother. The direct numinous experience was palpable and gave me sustenance to carry on the physical dimension of my beingness. She also shared messages with me which I was able to write down.

MESSAGES FROM DIVINE MOTHER BY
GAY LYNN WILLIAMSON-GRIGAS

I am the wisdom of the ages, asleep in the womb of
your being.

I awaken in you the remembrance of all mothers whose
wombs were the channels of life.

I have been hidden away in the cave of your uncon-
sciousness, in the dark places in the earth.

Always present yet not acknowledged, always available but unseen.

Now I am visiting your dreams, my energy stirring in your heart, my passion alive in you!

Let the message emerge in each person as it will. Follow it, follow the mystery.

GOING BEYOND MY PERSONAL EGO

Psychedelics have helped me to expedite the process by quickly facilitating me to go beyond my own ego-encapsulated flesh. In doing so, the healing, harmonizing, and light of the Spirit, has an opening and a channel to pour directly into my being. In my own experience with the sacred journeys using psilocybin, I have experienced freedom from the limitations of my personal self. I must admit, this is probably one of the most enjoyable factors, just getting beyond my own ego-bound self. In this state, I have a sense of unity and connection to something much greater than myself. It is a sense of pure being beyond my body and my senses. Although the vibrations and sensations are tangible in my body. I am in a state of extraordinary ethereal intelligence. The feeling is free and blissful.

REDUCING VALVE

Gary Lachman wrote in his book, *On Henri Bergson's Theory of the Mind and Cosmic Consciousness* that the brain's function for Henri Bergson was to act as a "reducing valve", limiting the amount of

"Reality" entering our consciousness. As Lachman wrote in his wonderful study of Bergson, "The brain is the organ of attention to life, and the part it plays is that of shutting out from consciousness all that is of no practical interest to us." Additionally, "Cosmic consciousness, then, can be seen as a perception of the world not limited by or filtered through the brain." So much may be filtered out for survival. So much more may be available. Psychedelics are a way to open the valve so to speak.

Aldous Huxley also observed the mind as a "reducing valve." He states, "To make biological survival possible, Mind at Large has to be funneled through the reducing valve of the brain and nervous system. What comes out at the other end is a measly trickle of the kind of consciousness that will help us to stay alive on the surface of this planet."

The funneling out of things in consciousness oftentimes eliminates much of the world from our conscious awareness. Michael Pollan describes it this way, "That stingy, vigilant security guard admits only the narrowest bandwidth of reality, a measly trickle of the kind of consciousness which will help us stay alive. It's really good at performing all those activities that natural selection values, like getting ahead, getting liked and loved, getting fed, getting laid. Keeping us on task, it is a ferocious editor of anything that might distract us from the work at hand, whether this means regulating our access to memories and strong emotions from within or news of the world without."

HOLDING A NEW PERSPECTIVE
LARGER THAN THE TRAUMA

Many people, through the psychedelic journey, achieve this non-ordinary state of transcendence and have a connection beyond their trauma. In fact, the trauma takes a back seat, a smaller bandwidth, may become a tiny speck rather than a log in the proverbial eye of the beholder. In this non-ordinary state, they connect with a power greater than themselves. The mystical connection appears to be a key component to healing and release from the captivity of the prison of trauma. What emerges is a part of us that can hold a new picture that is larger than the trauma. There is a capacity to be outside the jar of the trauma and look back at what is in the jar in a more detached yet conscious way. When we are trapped in the jar of the trauma it is hard to see the outside view of the jar.

MY PERSONAL MYSTICAL CONNECTION

For me, this mystical connection is my inner world, my interior abode, my inner castle. I am also connecting with my central power source. At times I am exploring the interior castle going over bridges, opening big wooden doors, discovering lush gardens, new trails and pathways, and investigating with curiosity, the rooms filled with light in my inner world. Some rooms have so much information to be shared, that I receive it as a cascade or download of files, pictures, images, information, and many symbols, into my mind.

At other times I feel a deep connection with nature and like a tree with my deepest roots going down into my own psyche and spirit. My tree trunk has its inner grounding and roots deep in my mystical connection to a larger presence and power, my mother Gaia, our Mother Earth. From this place, there is a sense of merging my small self with a greater Self. I am more aware of my connection to profound wisdom, an inner truth, the divine connection to my wholeness and my holiness. I am much larger spiritually than my small ego self and this awareness brings me comfort. In some way, I feel an internal alignment with something supernatural.

HEARING MY OWN INNER MESSAGES

In my mystical connection, there is also an experience of being in unity with my guides and teachers. This connection is very strong and I have developed these connections over many years. My experience with psychedelic medicines in this state of non-ordinary consciousness is where I can hear inner messages more clearly. I know my intuitive inner sensibilities and hear more clearly what my guides and teachers are saying to me.

Again, I can listen better in this non-ordinary state as I can easily move beyond the dissonance of my own ego, the machinations of my own ruminating thought loops, go past the ego chatter. I am in communion with my inner sphere. For me, this place is much less hectic than my ordinary consciousness. While in my inner realms I am more vibrantly in tune, I am sensing an infinite reality, an awareness of the everlasting touching into the eternal.

MY EXPERIENCE OF OCEANIC ONENESS

During my psychedelic medicine journey, there is a deep sense of oceanic oneness with myself and a profound love connection with others, the earth, and animals. When my husband is by my side sitting with me on my journey, I feel a love for him that is indescribable by words alone and brings tears to my eyes.

Love is experienced in a much more profound way with him on the journey. My husband and I share a passionate link between us as a depth of tenderness and devotion. Our relationship expands to touch into the deepest loyalty two people can share, which is vast in scope and measure. Again, mere sentences could not accurately describe these feelings. The sensitivity of connection is having a mystical spiritual quality beyond both of us and touches into the transcendent dimension. The word "bliss" comes close to describing the experience.

My oceanic connection with the earth and sky, the birds chirping and singing, all plants swaying and filled with life. My own dog is so spectacular as if he is speaking to me directly with a language I could understand and feel beyond words with just a look in his eyes. There is no separation, only allness and wholeness. With this comes a sense of awe and renewed sense of wonder. It is indescribably beautiful.

MY EXPERIENCE OF ENTERING KAIROS

In my psychedelic experiences of non-ordinary states, I am much less aware of time and space and it is more malleable. I can travel through the time-space continuum to the future and the past, and touch into multidimensional universes. I am fully aware that I am in my home, or wherever I may be, however, my home, my body, are like a base from which I could leave and then find my way back. The transcendence of time and space is noticeable. During my sacred journeys I am not in Kronos time anymore, the daily ticking away of minutes on the clock. Instead, I am in Kairos, which is deeper time, and the fullness of time of the expansive and numinous experience of non-ordinary time, the mystical experience the Greeks called Kairos.

There was a fine energetic thread of light and sound that kept me energetically connected to my body and my home base. At first, this being outside my ego-encapsulated body suit was a bit disconcerting. I was afraid to leave my body and my home, but I soon found it easier to leave it and then return.

I remembered how the shamans go to the underworld, the middle world, and the upper world and then return. I found it was like following a golden thread of sounds and subtle perceptions. At times I felt I was beyond this universe and visiting other beings in other realms and portal dimensions. In these realms, there seemed to be less restrictive patterns on the space-time boundaries. Particularly the sense of the eternal now touching into other dimensions of reality. In the everlasting realms, a minute can seem to linger and stretch forward, while hours can appear to pass in quick succession as a few seconds.

MY EXPERIENCE OF NUMINOSITY

The process of giving birth is related to Carl Jung's conception of "numinosity," in which he describes the aura of great light, and of great warmth that is attached to the archetypes when they become revealed directly in a non-ordinary state. Numinosity is the expression of great psychic intensity. As a result, in the moment of the psychedelic experience of non-ordinary consciousness, I know I am one with all life. The great paranormal intensity and the numinosity of the experience carry more weight and create a psychic imprint on my soul. It is very different from what happens in ordinary consciousness and makes a deeper life-changing impression. So, when a numinous non-ordinary state happens, it draws a larger concentration of psychic energy around it. So, in a sense, the awareness of connectedness is more dynamic and indelible.

MY PERSONAL BIRTHING WITH PSYCHEDELIC MEDICINE

On my own psychedelic journey, I often see a tunnel; it is a kind of birth canal. To experience myself as connected to the whole of creation. To see, feel, taste, touch the deep knowing that I am one with all life, all beingness now. To know that I can safely open to Divine Matrix. To open to the rebirth of myself and to recreate myself from within. My own connection to the creator/creatress is always there and always happening and endlessly creative. To be a conscious part of that creative dynamic. To experience the contentedness numinous oneness and spark of divinity within myself. To know with every fiber of my being the God-Goddess Head is real and constantly flowing and giving birth to itself perpetually through me. The Divine maternal womb of life manifests unendingly and eternally.

Here is a favorite poem that describes our existence, that is here but also where we have come from. It speaks of our soul search for true knowledge of the heart as we come into this life from another setting beyond this one. A wonderful way to conceive our physical and metaphysical birth.

IN ON SELF-KNOWLEDGE, KAHLIL GIBRAN
SPEAKS OF OUR SOUL BIRTH IN THIS WAY:

And a man said, Speak to us of Self-Knowledge.
And he answered, saying:
Your hearts know in silence the secrets of the days
and the nights.
But your ears thirst for the sound of your heart's knowledge.
You would know in words that which you have always
known in thought.
You would touch with your fingers the naked body
of your dreams.
And it is well you should.
The hidden well-spring of your soul must needs rise and
run murmuring to the sea;
And the treasure of your infinite depths would be revealed
to your eyes.
But let there be no scales to weigh your unknown treasure;
And seek not the depths of your knowledge with staff or
sounding line.
For self is a sea boundless and measureless.
Say not, "I have found the truth," but rather,
"I have found a truth."
Say not, "I have found the path of the soul." Say rather, "I
have met the soul walking upon my path."
For the soul walks upon all paths.
The soul walks not upon a line, neither does it grow like a reed.
The soul unfolds itself, like a lotus of countless petals.

–From The Prophet (Knopf, 1923)

EXPLORING MYSTICAL SOUL EXPERIENCES

The Carmelite nun and prominent Spanish mystic and religious reformer, Teresa of Avila, once said, "The soul is capable of much more than we can imagine. It is very important for any soul that practices prayer...not to hold itself back and stay in one corner. Let it walk through those dwelling places which are above, down below, and to the sides since God has given it such great dignity."

Explore your soul experience and look in every corner of your life, not just on occasion but every day, everywhere. The root word of psychology was formed by combining the Greek psyche, which means breath, principle of life, life, or soul, with logia which comes from the logos meaning speech or word or reason. So, in exploring our soul we give it meaning and breath by our own words and our own reason and our own exploration of its depth. Here are some other approaches:

- Meditate quietly and be open to ideas and feelings.

- Spend time in nature. Work in your garden. Feel oneness with all life.

- Read good poetry. Listen to quality music, especially classical music.

- Have a prayer life where you commune silently with God. Listen to the "still small voice" within you.

- Do drumming, chanting, dancing, yoga, tai chi.

- Put your hands over your heart when you lie down or meditate. Bless your heart and let your heart "speak" to you.

- Keep a life journal in which you write your innermost feelings.
- Do artwork: drawing, painting, sculpting.

Here are some questions you can ask yourself and explore:

THE OPENNESS OF THE SPIRITUAL LIFE BEYOND THE EGO

This truly requires an openness to understanding what lies beneath and beyond our ego. This requires a surrendering of what we think we know. Write a few of your thoughts on the following questions:

What is the nature of your being?

....
....
....
....

What is the nature of the universe?

....
....
....
....

How do we know what we know?

....
....
....
....

Where are you on your journey to discovering the nature of your being?

....

....

....

....

What is the nature of your own Inner Healer? How do you care for and nourish your life daily from this perspective?

....

....

....

....

Can you take the step away from prescribed beliefs into a new openness of what the metaphysical world wants to reveal to you and show you what lies beyond matter?

....

....

....

....

What can you do to deeply understand and wonder about the deeper wisdom and power that are a part of who you are?

....

....

....

....

How can you allow and open the way for more of your imprisoned splendor to be revealed?

....

....

....

....

What you see with your eyes open is only a part of the picture. Are you open to seeing with your eyes closed, the view of your inner landscape? Are you willing to explore how much more you can see with your eyes closed?

....

....

....

....

What do you think may happen when you look at your existence metaphysically? How does your awareness of yourself or others change or broaden metaphysically?

....

....

....

....

In your relationship with your inner world, how can you touch the most creative and regenerative part of your being, daily?

....

....

....

....

Are you paying attention to your mystical signs and signals?

....

....

....

....

Do you feel the awareness of the aliveness reflected in yourself and in all living creatures?

....

....

....

....

6

Ego Death and End-of-Life Distress

LIVING OUR DYING

So, we are all invited to enter this transpersonal dimension by facing our dying more consciously now. Helping to lead us into a transcendental dimension of existence to discover more of our identity beyond the physical body and the ego. Through dreams, rituals, and psychedelics, we enter this experience of transcendence in the body, and we come to terms with the problems of impermanence and our mortality. We can confront our fear of death overcome it and bring it into full conscious awareness of existential distress. In the process, we can experience our identity and release ourselves from the emotional and psychosomatic healing of suffering at the end of life.

FEAR OF DEATH

The end of life can bring some trepidation and fear for those who are not ready or prepared. This can be a terrifying time of life when facing our end-of-life journey. Michael Pollan, in his book, *How to*

Change Your Mind, shares on experimentation with psychedelics and those facing their dying. "The New York University, psilocybin trips take place in a treatment room carefully decorated to look more like a cozy den than a hospital suite."

Pollan goes on to describe his encounters with some of the therapists working with people approaching the end of their lives. "For the therapist, these questions are more than an academic interest." As Pollan chatted with Stephen Ross and Tony Bossis conducting the psilocybin journeys in this cozy NYU treatment room, he reported, "I was struck by their excitement verging in giddiness, at the results they were observing in their cancer patients—after a single guided psilocybin session."

COULD THIS BE FAKE?

At first, Ross could not believe what he was seeing:

I thought the first ten or twenty people were plants--that they must be faking it. They were saying things like, "I understand love is the most powerful force on the planet," or, "I had an encounter with my cancer, this black cloud of smoke."

People were journeying to the early parts of their lives and coming back with a profound new sense of things, and priorities. People who had been palpably scared of death--they lost their fear. The fact that a drug given once could have such an effect for so long is an unprecedented finding. We have never had anything like that in the psychiatric field.

RECALIBRATING THE WAY WE DIE

Pollan continues with his interview with Bossis, "As a palliative care specialist," Bossis shared, "I spend a lot of time with the dying. People don't realize how few tools we have in psychiatry to address existential distress."

Existential distress is what psychologists call the complex of depression, anxiety, and fear, common in people confronting a terminal diagnosis. "Xanax isn't the answer." If there is an answer, Bossis believes it is going to be more spiritual in nature than pharmacological. "So how do we explore this," he asks, "If it (psilocybin) can recalibrate how we die?"

PSYCHEDELIC DYING: ALDOUS HUXLEY

Huxley proposed that the fear of the experience of dying was really a function of the ego that saw that it was separate from something larger than itself and had no existence beyond the limited borders of the ego self. The ego somehow sensing itself as separate, became fearful. The psychedelic journey had the potential of opening one to the transcendent self. With this potential opening to the feeling of transcendence, there would no longer exist the fear and feeling of being separate and alone.

At the end of his own life, Huxley had instructed his wife, at the designated time, to inject him with LSD. On his deathbed, unable to speak because of laryngeal cancer, he wrote a note, "LSD, 100mg, intramuscular." His wife followed and did as her husband requested. At 11:20 a.m., with a second dose an hour later, Huxley died at the age of 69 years old, on November 22, 1963. Interesting that the media coverage of his death, along with the death of author C.S. Lewis on the very same day, was overshadowed by the assassination of President John F. Kennedy, less than seven hours before Huxley's death.

LETTING GO OF THE EGO

Michael Pollan interviewed Katherine MacLean, a former Johns Hopkins psychologist who worked with cancer patients having the psychedelic experience. MacLean reported:

> You're losing everything you know to be real, letting go of your ego and your body, and that process can feel like dying. Pollan continues, The experience brings the comforting news that there is something on the other side of that death—whatever it is, the "great plane of consciousness." Many described their experience of this transcendence as a plane of existence that is infinite and a place of pure love.

During non-ordinary states, there is a lifting of the veil to the possibility of new planes of awareness and a reassurance that there may be something greater than the ego self. This may be comforting to know the journey continues and there is continuity. There is something on the other side and we just might be in unity with the infinite.

THE COSMIC GAME

Stan Grof writes in his book *The Cosmic Game:*

People, who have during their lifetime experientially confronted birth and death and connected with the transpersonal dimension, have good reasons to believe that their physical demise will not mean the end of their existence. They have personally experienced in a very convincing way that their consciousness transcends the boundaries of their physical body, and it is capable of functioning independently of it.

Grof continues:

As a result, they tend to see death as a transition into a different state of existence and an awe-inspiring adventure in consciousness rather than a final defeat and annihilation. Naturally, this attitude can substantially change the approach to death and the experience of dying. In addition, people who are involved in deep self-exploration have the opportunity to gradually come to terms with many difficult aspects of their unconscious that we otherwise have to deal with in the final period of our life.

DYING BEFORE DYING

In the shamanic traditions, Grof describes the role of the death and rebirth experiences. Interestingly this was also a dynamic and powerful scene in the movie, *The Black Panther,* where the death and rebirth initiation is played out as a ceremonial burial. Once given the elixir and then "buried" the Black Panther visits his father and his ancestors in the other dimensions.

Stan Grof writes:

By undergoing death and rebirth in their initiatory crisis, shamans lose their fear of death and become familiar and comfortable with its experiential territory. As a result, they can later visit this realm on their own terms and mediate similar experiences for others. In the mysteries of death and rebirth, which are widespread in the Mediterranean area and other parts of the ancient world, initiates experienced a profound symbolic confrontation with death. In this process, they lost the fear of death and developed an entirely new set of values and strategies for life.

Again, Grof writes:

The shamans have personally experienced in a very convincing way that their consciousness transcends the boundaries of their physical body and is capable of functioning independently of it. In the West, it also points us toward the core of the Christian religious tradition which is the death and resurrection of Jesus and his constant message of "Do not be afraid, I am with you always, even to the end of the age" from the Gospel of Matthew.

EXISTENTIAL DISTRESS

Existential distress at the end of life is a common theme for many people. Pollen shares:

> The whole question of meaning is central to the approach of the NYU therapists and is especially helpful in understanding the experience of cancer patients on psilocybin. For many of these patients, a diagnosis of terminal cancer constitutes, among other things, a crisis of meaning: Why me? Why have I been singled out for this fate? Is there any sense to life and the universe?

This may be the precise place the psychedelic medicine can help the most. "Under the weight of this existential crisis, one's horizon shrinks, one's emotional repertoire contracts and one's focus narrows as the mind turns in on itself, shutting out the world. Loops of rumination and worry come to occupy more of one's mental time and space, reinforcing habits of thought it becomes more difficult to escape." Psychedelic medicine operates as a catalysis for a new view, an entrance to another dimension beyond what currently exists.

Pollen reported, "Temporarily disabling the ego, psilocybin opens a new field of psychological possibility, symbolized by the death and rebirth reported by many of the patients interviewed." At first, Pollen reported, "The falling away of the self feels threatening, but as one can let go and surrender, powerful and usually positive emotions flow in—along with formerly inaccessible memories and sense impressions and meanings. And what comes through that opening for many people, in a great flood, is love."

DEATH DOES NOT END RELATIONSHIPS

My mom died before my dad. It was a big loss for us all, especially for my dad. He had to adjust to not having my mom around after 55 years of marriage. I have had many goodbyes over the last ten years of my life. I have grieved for the loss of my aunts, uncles, cousins, friends, and even many friends and clients who have made their passage to the next dimensions of life and experiences.

Soon after my mom passed, she would visit me in my dreams. Visitations by my mom were a special treat. One night, very soon after she passed, she came to me in a dream and showed me the new place where she lived. It was all purple, her favorite color. During her memorial service, a few weeks after her passing, the minister mentioned that my mom was now happy, and her place was ready and waiting for her that her room was all purple! It was strangely comforting as I had never shared with the minister about my dream of Mom being in her purple room.

Intuitively or in some way, it was a message from my mom, whom he had never met before. When we enter non-ordinary states of consciousness with others, we can be informed in magnificent ways beyond what we can see, feel, taste, and touch in this dimension. The time of death and making this transition seems to be an opening in a way, like a portal or bridge between this dimension and the next.

PACKING DAD'S SUITCASE FOR HIS JOURNEY HOME

A couple of years later, when my dad was closer to his time of death and was passing on from this life, my mom came to me again in a dream. This time, she was packing my dad's suitcases with all his clothes. She smiled at me as she was busy getting all his things together. I knew intuitively that she was getting ready to meet him and was picking up all his stuff for his journey home. This was her message to me. I shared the dream with my sister as Dad's health was beginning to fail. It was only a matter of weeks when my sister told me Mom had come to get Dad and take him home and that he had passed away. It gave me some comfort to be able to conceptualize the loss of my parents in this way.

The loss of my dad was a big one for me. My dad was my herald. My dad was the one who introduced me to dreams, psychology, and the understanding of the mystical and metaphysical realms. My dad showed me how to make my connection with the Divine Mind, Universal Mind, Creative intelligence, my Inner Healer, and God within. I am forever grateful to my mom and dad for all they shared.

THE SUDDEN DEATH OF MY HUSBAND: NO GOODBYES

After fourteen years of marriage, my husband David dropped dead following a massive heart attack. He had gone home to run an errand. Our real estate agent discovered him while showing our home to a prospective client. When the real estate agent came in to show our home, he thought my husband was sleeping with his head down at the dining room table. I was called while at the church where I was working, to be informed that they had found him unresponsive at home. The church staff and friends gathered in my office, and we prayed together. My real estate agent called EMS and stayed on the phone as they arrived and worked to revive him. Eventually, the agent said to me, "I am sorry darling, he has gone; they could not bring him back." My husband simply went home to run an errand, sat down at the dining room table, and passed out of this life.

Back at my office at the church, I heard the news, stood up, and passed out, right there; the shock was overwhelming. One moment, just a couple of hours before, we had been sharing lunch together and a quick kiss goodbye, and I said, "I will see you at the prayer group later." A couple of hours later, he was gone.

NO LAST WORDS

The hard part was, there was no goodbye, no closure, no last words, no hugs; he was gone in an instant. I was in a daze. The night before, we had seen a funny movie at the theatre, come home, had some dinner, and he was watching one of his favorite old movies on TV, *Bullitt,* with Steve McQueen and the crazy car chase through the streets of San Francisco. He was so happy.

I sensed, in some ways, that he was becoming weaker. Only a few months before, I had dreadful dreams and woke up crying because I had seen that he was going to pass away. The dream was so clear. I did not want him to die. I shared this dream with him. I was weeping in his arms, telling him to do whatever he needed to do to keep on living and thriving. He was comforting me the best he could. I did not want our time together to end. He died at the height of his career success, we just had a new book come out, we traveled to Hawaii for a conference and book tour, he received an award from his peers, and he was so happy. Then it was over.

FIRST NIGHT AFTER DAVID DIED,
HE CAME TO SPEAK TO ME

One of the women who worked with me at the church stayed all night the first night. I was not tired; I was in this strange, numb, alert place that was painful and uncomfortable. Finally, lying in our bed, smelling my husband's pillow, I fell asleep for a few hours.

When I awoke, it was my husband's voice that woke me. He said my name, "Gay, get up." It was just before dawn and still somewhat dark. He urged me, "Get up and look out the window." So, I got up and walked to the window. He spoke to me as if he were standing in the room next to me and said, "Look out the window." It was dark, but the sun was just starting to rise over the horizon from our home on Dildo Island on Miami Beach. I could see the sky beginning to light up with the hint of dawn.

My husband spoke to me again, *"It is not death, but dawn. Look!"* and just as he said it, the sun rose and came shining over the horizon. I felt an incredible inner warmth and peace.

A slight smile came to my face because David was with me, sharing a part of one of our favorite poems that we had used many times at funerals and memorial services we officiated, written by our friend James Dillet Freeman. He came to say goodbye to me and give me a clear message that there is life and a new dawn beyond what we think of as death. There is no death, only new dawns, and new horizons. And we were ever one beyond the veil, always and forever. Here is the poem he recited the line from:

The Traveler

He has put on invisibility.
Dear Lord, I cannot see—
But this I know, although the road ascends
And passes from my sight,
That there will be no night;
That You will take him gently by the hand
And lead him on
Along the road of life that never ends,
And he will find *it is not death but dawn.*
I do not doubt that You are there as here,
And You will hold him dear.
Our life did not begin with birth,
It is not of the earth;
And this that we call death, it is no more
Than the opening and closing of a door—
And in Your house how many rooms must be
Beyond this one where we rest momently.
Dear Lord, I thank You for the faith that frees,
The love that knows it cannot lose its own;
The love that, looking through the shadows, sees
That You and he and I are ever one!

COMFORT OF SAYING GOODBYE

I was able to say goodbye. And David came to me to say goodbye after his death. I was deeply comforted to hear his voice and his message. I was deeply grateful for him to come to me and say, as clearly as he possibly could, that he was fine. He wanted me to know there was no death and separation as we typically think of with the end of life, only a new dawn. So, he came to share his love and comfort with me.

I lay back down in our bed with a different kind of peace. I was still in shock, but there was some healing, some tiny bit of coming to terms with the loss, some connection that made me feel more reassured that we would always be connected on the spiritual dimension by our love. He crossed the bridge between the two worlds that always exist between dimensions and said goodbye. I was learning to cross that bridge back and forth as well within my dreams.

David was so incredibly thoughtful, and it was immensely healing for me. It was his visitation that helped to give me the strength to move on over the months that followed. In so many ways, his speaking with me briefly that morning at dawn helped me to make closure.

ANCESTRAL CONNECTIONS-KEEPING IN TOUCH WITH THOSE PASSED ON

With some family members who are open and receptive, these conversations can be extremely helpful before they make their transition from one life to the next. The idea is that, clearly, there is a way to stay in touch. I had these honest and open conversations with my Uncle Bob about staying in touch and told him that I had conversations with his mother and sisters, who had passed on during my dreams. Then unexpectedly and suddenly, Uncle Bob died. It was extremely hard on our family when my uncle passed, and his son Mike and his wife Judy had been with him just before he died. So, I got the painful call from my cousin

Mike that the EMS had come to the house. They took him to the hospital, but they could not revive him, and he had passed away. His death was a big shock for us all. That night I had a dream, and in the dream, I was with Uncle Bob and Mike.

In the dream, my cell phone rang, and I answered it; it was Uncle Bob! He said, "Hi, this is Uncle Bob." I was so thrilled to hear his voice. In our family, whenever anyone was traveling anywhere, we would call to say that we had arrived safely. So, this was a long-standing tradition in our family. So, in the dream, I asked, "How are you?" And he says, "I am fine, I am doing okay," with his happy laughter, which was always such a joy to hear. I said, "Mike told me you died?" And Uncle Bob said, "No, I am doing good!" And I say, "I am so happy to hear this, and can't wait to tell Mike and the others in the family."

It was a brief conversation in the dream, but so powerful and deeply comforting. My Uncle Bob kept his word and called after he died to let us all know he was "doing okay, and he had arrived safely."

What became abundantly clear to me is that consciousness does not end or die. The body passes away, but what makes us who we are continues to exist beyond our body experience. We are truly immortal beings. One night, I received this beautiful message in my dream, "All of us are immortals, some of us just recognize this now!" The clarity is in the recognition of this now. Psychedelics and dreams help in many ways to open the pathway for this clarity.

OPEN TO THE LIFE OF SPIRIT

As Mircea Eliade had indicated from his study of the paradigms in religious experiences, through non-ordinary states, we are a being "open to the life of spirit," and in doing so, our existence is no longer perceived as separate. If our journey and our existence is perceived as separate through the lenses of the ego, we become fearful prisoners in a prison cell we have created for ourselves. Through the psychedelic journey and dream work, we may be holding the keys of transcendence in our own hands. Through the voyage, we are prepared for the transition from this life moving forward. By connecting to the transcendent part of ourselves in non-ordinary states of consciousness, we have touched our God Self, that "one mind," and we can know and perceive things far beyond our conscious mind's limitations. Non-ordinary states send a powerful message to our deeper self, our spiritual self, and our inner healer. By doing so, it connects us with our infinite Self and in spirit with one another unceasingly beyond the dimension that we call death. Dreams and visitations are a way to experience our connectedness to the dimension beyond. What we call death is really a bridge between dimensions that we can learn to cross.

THERAPEUTIC POWERS OF LSD

Amanda Feilding is the Founder and Director of the Beckley Foundation. Amanda has been called the "hidden hand" behind the renaissance of psychedelic science, and her contribution to global drug policy reform. Amanda was first introduced to LSD in the mid-1960s, at the height of the first wave of scientific research into psychedelics. Amanda was impressed by LSD's capacity to initiate mystical states of consciousness and heighten creativity, she quickly recognized its transformative and therapeutic power.

Inspired by her experiences, Amanda began studying the mechanisms underlying the effects of psychedelic substances and dedicated herself to exploring ways of harnessing their potential to cure sickness and enhance well-being. Through her leadership of the Beckley Foundation's Science Program, Amanda has initiated groundbreaking research and has coauthored over fifty scientific articles published in peer-reviewed journals.

REGENERATING BRAIN ACTIVITY
AND END-OF-LIFE DEMENTIA

I had the pleasure of meeting Amanda at the ICPR conference in the Netherlands in 2022. She showed a picture of a ninety-plus-year-old woman in the final stages of dementia, barely able to speak or recognize family members. After the family gave permission, the woman was administered a micro-dosing of LSD. The woman became more animated and began having recognizable conversations and access to memories long forgotten. In Amanda's words, she believes that "LSD is the Queen" of all substances and may have the possibility of regenerating brain activity in ways we are only beginning to understand. She is interested in studying brain regeneration, particularly in dementia-related cases with individuals.

In Amanda's role as the co-director of the Beckley/Imperial Psychedelic Research Program, she helped generate the world's first images of the brain on LSD, one of her long-standing ambitions. Amanda continues to bridge the divide between science and drug policy. Her pioneering psychedelic research is providing evidence to fuel a fair debate on drug policy reform. Such reform will, in turn, allow for research on currently prohibited psychedelic substances to flourish, uninhibited by regulatory obstructions. We stand on the shoulders of giants, and so then we can see further than the giants. Amanda Feilding is a giant and has helped us all see more clearly into a new future of brain health and well-being. Imagine what we might tap into as we understand more about dementia and how to enhance brain function as we age.

CREATIVELY BEING BORN AGAIN AND AGAIN

We developed in our mother's womb for nine months, and then we are born out of the opportunity for greater development and expression. The life experience in the womb ends, but it leads naturally to other possibilities. Development in the womb is followed by increased life opportunities. This is the way the Creative life and our process work for our entire life and beyond.

In this lifetime, I see it as actually being born again and again as I pass through various stages of life and development and experiences. Although I have changed dramatically in many ways, I am still "me." When I leave this body, I trust there is further life expression, development, and work to do. I believe that life is abundant and limitless. All of us are immortals on an immortal journey into new life.

We are living our eternal life right now. So, the question then, for me, is not, "Where will I spend eternity?" But, "Am I living fully in the eternal now?'

Salutation To The Dawn

Look to this day,
for it is Life, the very life of life,
Within its brief span,
Lie all the Verities and realities
of your existence.
The Bliss of Growth.
The Glory of Action.
The Splendor or Beauty.
For yesterday is but a dream
and tomorrow is but a Vision
but today well lived makes every yesterday
a dream of happiness
and every tomorrow a vision of Hope.
Look well therefore To this day.

–The Sanskrit

The important realization for me is that life is not measured in terms of length but of quality. Perhaps "Eternal Life" refers to the quality of our life and not the quantity of life. Perhaps it is not how long we live but how *well* we live. Oliver Wendell Holmes once said, "To be seventy years young is sometimes more cheerful and hopeful than to be forty years old." We can be more fully alive, alert, and enthusiastic about life and living no matter what our chronological age may be.

George Bernard Shaw wrote:

"I rejoice in life for its own sake. Life is not a brief candle to me. It is a sort of splendid torch which I have got hold of for a moment, and I want to make it burn as brightly as possible before handing it on to future generations."

QUESTIONS TO EXPLORE:

What do you think about your own death and dying?

....

....

....

....

What have you experienced when other people you know have died? Is there still a connection?

....

....

....

....

Have you experienced ancestral and family or friend visitations after death?

....

....

....

....

How might psychedelics help with end-of-life distress?

....

....

....

....

Is there a possibility of seeing your own death as a transition to a different state or transpersonal dimension of being?

....

....

....

....

How do you see psychedelic medicines helping with your own fears around death and dying?

....

....

....

....

Triune
Pathway Three:
Rituals

Chapter Seven details some of the lessons and insights on connecting with one another in the sanctuary of a group or community of people. We often heal best in a group of caring people. Being in a community has a deepening effect on everyone. Important guidelines are shared for group work so the boundaries are clear and everyone can prepare for the best group experiences and feel safe and supported.

Chapter Eight explores how using psychedelics, dreams, and rituals in addiction treatment, and entering non-ordinary states of consciousness can make a significant difference for people in recovery.

There are inner transformations and insights I explore through the stories of people who had life-changing experiences while in treatment for addictions. I believe we are only just beginning to see the ways we might incorporate the use of non-addictive psychedelics into a vibrant program of recovery, as did the co-founder of AA, Bill W.

Chapter Nine presents my fun and effective therapeutic tools based on Cognitive Behavioral Therapy (CBT), which is vital to processing the client's triggers and understating family of origin issues that are often repeated over generations. Psychotherapy is a vital component in effective psychedelic-assisted therapy. You will have detailed tools you can use personally and that you can

PSYCHEDELICS DREAMS & RITUALS

teach your clients to help them understand how to handle their personal triggers. There is step-by-step learning on how to hold on to personal power and peace of mind.

Chapter Ten concludes with rituals of healing, including the best of rituals and ceremonies from Transformative Rituals: Celebrations for Personal Growth. These are offered in detail to be creatively used by those needing fresh ideas to enhance the set and setting for healing rituals and ceremonies. Included are some favorites, such as the Burning Bowl Ceremony, Spiritual Naming Ceremony, Inner Mapping, Heart-to-Heart, and Phoenix Rising.

7

Relationship with Self and Community

NEW KIND OF COMMUNION

The psychedelic experience is a different kind of communion. Humanistic. Experiential. Communion between people in a community. Not drinking wine or eating bread but touching and experiencing our spiritual natures with each other. The love feast, which communion originally was, is exchanging love and affirming love. Rituals, psychedelic plant ceremonies, and healing rites of passage in a gathering allow for the experience of the community. The experience can be very intimate and uplifting as people are empowered through the community ritual to affirm and support each other.

EXPERIENCE OF COMMUNITY IS KEY

A community is a body of people having common interests and organizations. Ritual has the deepening effect of giving a sense of belonging to a community. My experience and the experience I have shared with others collaborate a transcending of the personality into the levels beyond and a deeper sense of relating and participation. The sharing of power on an equal basis is key to the experience of ritual in the community.

LOVE AND COMMUNITY CONNECTION

Love is an emotion, but it is also a real power. Our lives are shaped by the way we use our love power or ability to share in loving relationships in the community with others. To love is to live! The Scottish scientist and minister, Henry Drummond, said in his classic little book, *Love: The Greatest Thing in the World,* "You will find as you look back upon your life that the moments that stand out, the moments when you have really lived, are the moments when you have done things in a spirit of love."

There is a dynamic flow of life expressed through us. We call this life force by religious and scientific names: God, energy, prana, chi. This life force seeks to express itself fully and freely through us and as us. We free up or maximize the life flow by love, being loving, and being loved. To love is to be in the flow of life, in the circulation of life, in the abundance of life.

The Dalai Lama has said that his religion is summed up in one word: kindness. He is following the steps of Gautama Buddha, whose teachings and example are centered on compassion. Love, kindness, compassion, and all ways of describing the flow of love. George Bernard Shaw once said, "The opposite of love is not hate, it is indifference." So, love and particularly caring and support from a community of people, nourish and uplift us. Smiley Blanton, MD, writes, "Love is the immortal flow of energy that nourishes, extends, and preserves. Its eternal goal is life."

THE HEALING POWER OF A LOVING GROUP

The twelve-step groups are a community of people concerned with sharing the spiritual path of recovery. Going to a twelve-step meeting can be an experience of being in a field of energy and community that is healing. In the meetings, there can be a sharing of unconditional acceptance, something rarely experienced outside of the meetings for the person in recovery. It takes a willingness to attend a meeting and step into a circle of people who accept without judgment because they know and have walked in the same shoes.

David Hawkins writes about how our thoughts have a certain electromagnetic field:

Thoughts have a certain electromagnetic energy form. When we sit in the presence of people who have solved life problems that we are confronting, their inner accomplishment influences us non-verbally so that our lower-level energy is replaced by a higher thought form. That higher thought form sees the problem as an excellent opportunity. What we saw as a loss before the meeting, now we see as a gain because of that nonverbal transmission. The facts have not changed, but how we view the situation has changed because our level of consciousness shifted. The shift occurred not because of the words spoken but by being in the presence of the aura of loving people whose energy field carries the higher wisdom. Simply put, we are either positively or negatively influenced by the company we keep. It is unlikely that we will overcome a problem if we choose to be in the company of others who have the same problem.

GUIDELINES FOR COMMUNITY
RITUALS AND CEREMONIES

....

1. **Let people choose whether to participate.**

   They can say "yes" or "no" to any ritual or psychedelic
   medicine ceremony experience, they must be well-in-
   formed and provide written consent. Participants are
   not obligated to answer why they might not want to do a
   certain ritual or ceremony. If at any point a group member
   opts out, it is okay, accept this without questions. We very
   seldom have a situation where a person does not want to
   participate fully, but it does occur sometimes. However, it
   is important that participants agree to stay until the end
   of the ritual or ceremony for safety reasons. Respect the
   rights and needs of everyone.

2. **Stress group support**

   Participation in the rituals and psychedelic medicine ceremonies gives people the opportunity to share in the power
   of love. We need to be honest and open with others and
   ourselves. If we truly do this, our honesty will be for the
   purpose of love. Some people will open for the first time,
   and this is a very tender and vulnerable space. Be gentle with
   one another. What is said in the group stays in the group
   and confidentiality is an important part of building trust.

3. **Learning and transformation by doing**

   In some instances, as the facilitator you will need to
   observe so you can give feedback; in other instances, you
   will have the opportunity to join in the ritual experience

and participate fully. As you share, participate, or facilitate the ritual and the community, be as present as possible. When you are the facilitator in a psychedelic medicine journey, it is your responsibility and essential that you monitor the safety of each person.

4. **Ask people to speak in the first person**
    So often, people talk about themselves in a veiled, unaware fashion. For instance, "When you have been closed up for a long time and are afraid of saying the wrong thing, it is difficult to walk in here and make some big changes." That person is not talking about "you" but about herself or himself. By using "I" when speaking of my experience I increase the potential for transformative experiences. Remind people of this and notice the change it makes as people "own what they are saying." Model this same "first person" perspective, as you are sharing as well.

5. **Keep people focused on the immediate ritual or ceremony**
    If they start talking about situations outside of the group, or other psychedelic journeys in other places with other people, bring them back to the present moment. The group may get distracted, off track, and start making comparisons. Be sure the group does not get into advising, taking sides, or solving others' problems. Do not let people stray too far from the here and now. Growth is in the present. Be here now!

6. **Treat people with love and respect, be firm and motivating when needed**

This is a delicate area because you want the group to be active and motivated, and this can be done by sharing a certain amount of your leadership and spontaneity. At the same time, you need to stay in the facilitator role and create gentle boundaries when needed, to carry out the ritual and psychedelic medicine ceremony and make sure that all the people in the group get a chance to fully engage and participate.

7. **Make sure everyone feels a part and can see and hear well**

If possible, keep circles small so all can hear. In larger groups, be sure there is adequate amplification of your voice so everyone hears the directions. Some people feel left out if they are not clear on what they are supposed to do. Make the balance between group and individual attention when needed.

8. **Start and end the group with reading or meditation.**

The opening may be given by you or someone else in the group. You may want to ask others to participate in this part of the opening ritual process. The closing at the end of each ritual or ceremony can be done by people just speaking a word or some brief thought they have. You may want to sing or chant at the beginning or end. People may get together in a closing huddle or "the spiral." The spiral is a chain of people joined together with their arms around shoulders or arms linked together standing in a loose spiral. Passing a talking stick with the option to share is a straightforward way to open and close the ritual space.

DISCLOSURE AND HONESTY IN COMMUNITY

The sharing part in group and community is also a kind of ritual. There is no doubt there is a strong psychological effect when you share things with other people. It is the cathartic effect that is well documented, whether you are talking about the Catholic confession, group therapy, psychoanalysis, or anything else. The sharing itself is a ritual.

I have experienced community sacred space, which I think accelerates the process. When using a psychedelic or non-ordinary state, it requires a lot of trust. But in many cases, people are so ready to have the experience it does not even occur to them that trust is an essential component. They just wanted to do it. Creating trust and holding the container for trust is an important part of holding sacred space.

Through entering non-ordinary states with the assisted by ritual and psychedelic medicines, there is a deepening of direct experience of the community or group. Also, the ability to access and express parts of the self that are not readily available in normal social conventions. So, in the context of the community and sacred space, access to all parts of the self are welcome and it is healthy and healing to express all the parts of themselves more freely. The sense of belonging and connecting to a group or community is a healing experience.

DEEPER LEVELS OF RELATING IN COMMUNITY

The ritual experience really helps to dissolve layers of personality that can separate us at times. Like walls or partitions between us, ritual in the community can help melt away the walls and disintegrate the perceived barriers and boundaries between us. One of my friends described it this way, "I think that the ritual work really helped dissolve those layers of personality and bring us to a different level of appreciation of one another. And a different level of relating to one another."

HEART-TO-HEART

During the Heart-To-Heart Ritual we pass around a small stuffed heart, we learn to leave the headspace and all our overthinking, and enter more fully into the heart space, speak from the heart, and share from the heart the secrets of our heart with one another. Only the person with the heart is allowed to speak. All others will listen with love and give the person their full attention. The person speaking can share whatever feelings come to mind.

The heart continues around the circle as many times as necessary. It is okay for people in the circle to pass on sharing. When no one has anything more to say, the sharing is concluded. The purpose is to maximize the expression of feelings, not to give a chronological rundown of current life events. As each person shares there is no comment about judging or analyzing what anyone else in the group has said. The key is to have honest expression and undivided attention.

THE HEART-TO-HEART COMMITMENT:

(Can be shared as an opening to the circles)
I commit myself to speaking from my heart during this time of sharing. I agree to be honest with myself and others. I also make every effort to listen intently, looking directly at the person with the heart who is speaking. I will help to create an atmosphere of trust, security, and peace where we can feel safe in reaching our own hearts and communicating Heart-To-Heart. I will honor and keep confidential all that is shared and never use it against the person or as gossip later. I make this commitment in the belief that love is the greatest thing in the world and can heal, uplift, harmonize, prosper, and bring peace.

EXPLORING COMMUNITY RITUALS FOR YOURSELF, QUESTIONS TO CONSIDER:

Do you have a sense of community connections that are meaningful to you?

....
....
....
....

Does your culture encourage you to connect with rituals and stories in a larger community sense?

....
....
....
....

Do you feel a loss of community and a loss of connection that is needing to be filled in your life in some way?

....

....

....

....

At its best, what could a loving, safe, and trusting community provide for you?

....

....

....

....

In the community rituals you have participated in, is there a connection to the transcendent or spiritual dimensions?

....

....

....

....

Describe what you would like to experience in a community of people sharing a psychedelic experience together.

....

....

....

....

What would it take to create a set and setting in a community of people for you to achieve this transcendent connection to others?

....

....

....

....

8

Rituals and Recovery

RITUALS OF INITIATION IN RECOVERY

The twelve-steps are a ritual in their own way, the progression through the steps. The meetings are group community rituals of sharing stories and entering healing consciousness with one another on the journey to sobriety is transformational. The meetings are guided by rules and customs. Most meetings have a chair and are highly ritualized exchanges with lots of respect for the individual talking, with no cross talk.

Addiction thrives and lives in isolation. The awareness of the power of the group and community is an important ingredient in the healing process. Combine that with some gut-level honesty and storytelling and you have the recipe for healing. It is storytelling within the community and relationship building that is key. Each person's healing is affirmed, validated, and recognized by those in the group that have been on the path of recovery for some time.

The group can be a place of experiencing a non-ordinary state of consciousness as each person reveals themselves within the safety of the meeting, like a sacred circle of caring. Not every meeting is always uplifting. However, there can be a larger presence felt, as in "where two or more are gathered in my name," the Great Spirit, the God of your choosing and your naming is present. The "I Am" beingness is during the circle. The group can be, and is for many, an extended family and the first sober family they ever had. In the group is a shared meaning and purpose to stay sober one more day.

TRANSFORMING THE WAY WE DO TREATMENT

Today we have the potential for a new paradigm. The use of transformative rituals and psychedelics in recovery is supported by both new and old research, giving renewed hope for entering the treatment experience in a fresh way. The fact is that the Twelve-Step Recovery program is a ritual process. *The Big Book: The Basic Text for Alcoholics Anonymous* states:

> Rarely have we seen a person fail who has thoroughly followed our path. "Our path" is a well-documented and highly structured form of ritual that has led thousands of people into a balanced and healthy life. Ritual is the most important factor in recovery. The addicted person already has many unhealthy rituals going, and the application of the rituals in AA can lead to stabilization and life-enhancing behaviors.

Although little talked about, it is well documented that Bill W. had his first spiritual psychedelic experience after being given Belladonna Cure in a hospital while being detoxed and treated for his alcoholism. His spiritual vision was the turning point of his life. Many years later Bill Wilson continued to experiment with LSD to overcome a continuing depression that was debilitating.

PARADOXICAL USING PSYCHEDELICS
TO OVERCOME ADDICTIONS?

We are only beginning to see the ways we might incorporate the use of non-addictive psychedelics into a vibrant program of recovery. This may seem paradoxical to use a psychedelic drug to help overcome another drug. Not necessarily when you understand addiction is sometimes defined as "spiritual bankruptcy," often characterized as being an emptiness or hole in the soul. Addictions have devastating consequences. The addicted person is trying to fill an inner emptiness with anything and everything.

In the end, there is just the experience of being sick and tired of being sick and tired. Never really getting any alleviation of the internal pain and suffering. While using ever-increasing amounts of drugs and alcohol to anesthetize the pain of emptiness.

SPIRITUAL BANKRUPTCY

Simply said, addiction is spiritual bankruptcy. And a spiritual malady needs a spiritual response. The experience of psychedelic medicine opened Bill Wilson. This psychedelic medicine became a catalyst for recovery for the co-founder of AA. In effect using a non-ordinary state of consciousness with the Belladonna Cure to help enter and change a highly dysfunctional non-ordinary state of consciousness, his alcoholism, into something more functional and life-affirming. People suffering from an addiction, who are "willing," can choose to travel a similar transformational pathway for spiritual and psychological healing through their own psychedelic rebirth and have new hope for their own recovery.

THE CONVERSION EXPERIENCE

....

One of the hallmarks of the experience of spiritual conversion was first introduced by Dr. Carl Jung, which may seem strange to some, but it is not because Jung had played a critical role in the formation of the fellowship. In the late 1920s an investment banker and former senator from Rhode Island, Rowland Hazard, was sinking deeper into his alcoholism and had tried everything. According to letters written between Hazard and his cousin, Pulitzer prizewinning poet Leonard Bacon, who was himself a patient of Dr. Jung's, recommended that his cousin go to see Dr. Jung as a last-ditch effort to save him. Hazard did well for several months while working with Dr. Jung, but then relapsed on a trip to Africa. During his second round of analysis with Dr. Jung, he told Hazard he was a chronic alcoholic and there was nothing more that psychiatry or medicine could do for him. Dr. Jung went on to give one glimmer of hope and said "that occasionally alcoholics could recover after experiencing some type of religious conversion, however, the recoveries attributed to a life-changing vital spiritual experience were relatively rare."

Dr. Carl Jung was not a stranger to religious experiences, having had a father and other uncles as clergy. Additionally, his mother was a spiritual woman and shared with her son that she had visions in the night where she was visited by spirits and had the gift of second sight and seeing more deeply beyond the physical into what we would perhaps call the mystical or metaphysical dimensions. Dr. Jung also worked as a young intern in a medical school, treating many alcoholics and alcohol-related problems.

HAVING A SPIRITUAL EXPERIENCE

....

This spiritual experience was a very unusual remedy and having that prognosis shook-up Hazard, who then returned to find fellowship in the Oxford Group, a Christian evangelical movement active in Europe and the United States from the 1920s to the 1930s. The association and fellowship that Hazard felt and experienced with the Oxford Group, proved the spiritual conversion experience for Hazard that Dr. Jung had talked about. Hazard stopped drinking and devoted his life to being of service through the Oxford Group to give hope and inspiration to others who were sick and suffering.

Hazard and a few other members from the Oxford Group were vacationing in Vermont in 1934 when they ran into an old friend, Edwin "Ebby" Thacher, who was a lifelong alcoholic, who went to jail several times and was on the verge of being institutionalized. The three Oxford Group members gathered up their friend Thacher and he was released in their care. Through prayer, reading the Bible, and the fellowship of the group, he was able to finally sustain sobriety.

After months of sobriety, Thacher went to visit one of his old drinking buddies with whom he had drank with for over twenty years, Bill Wilson. Thatcher shared his story with Wilson and explained Dr. Jung's message of a vital spiritual experience. He shared with Wilson how the Oxford Group had a way of helping you confess your character defects, admit defeat, and accept help from a "Higher Power." The reason he was there with Wilson was part of the program, as well as to be of service to others, and this was part of his restitution and staying sober as well.

Wilson continued to drink but finally decided to go to Calvary Church in Manhattan to see for himself and visit Thacher there, he was drunk when he arrived. Thatcher gave him some coffee and a bowl of beans to help him sober up and Wilson sat and heard the message. There must have been something that struck a chord because Wilson went home and told his wife he was going to quit drinking. Wilson was then admitted for detox to Town's Hospital for Drug and Alcohol Addiction in Manhattan. While in the hospital Wilson felt deeply depressed and he prayed and pleaded to God for help. "I'll do anything! Anything at all! If there be a God, let him show himself!" Wilson reported that the entire room was filled with light, and he described an ecstasy feeling, "A new world of consciousness" and an experience of "God and His word." That was the last time Bill Wilson ever drank alcohol. Wilson spent the rest of his life seeking this spiritual awakening and renewal.

While on a business trip to Akron, Ohio, Wilson found himself on shaky ground and reached out to a local physician, Dr. Bob Smith. The two men were deeply connected by their desire to stay sober and had long and deep conversations on how this takes place in a person's life. Wilson stayed at Dr. Bob Smith's home and while there at his home, Smith relapsed and started drinking again. Wilson was there to help his new friend and the last date that Dr. Bob Smith took a drink was June 10, 1935, the date celebrated as the anniversary of AA's founding. By 1939 the two friends had separated from the Oxford Group and the Fellowship of AA became an independent entity.

In 1961 after years of sobriety, Bill Wilson wrote to Dr. Carl Jung, he and other members of AA had read Jung's *Modern Man in Search of a Soul.* In the letter Wilson told Jung, "Your words really carried authority because you seemed to be neither wholly a theologian nor a pure scientist. Therefore, you seemed to stand with us in that no-man's land that lies between the two...You spoke a language of the heart that we could understand." The powerful combination of the therapeutic process and the spiritual dimension and love was what Jung, Wilson, and Dr. Bob put together. There is a legacy of spirituality and compassion with the psychological therapeutic process for inner healing working all together. It is the integration of spirituality with human health together. We have Dr. Carl Jung to thank for building the bridge between the two.

ADDRESSING THE SPIRITUAL MALADY

In my own experience working with hundreds of people, this is the way that appears to work the best to address the spiritual malady and spiritual bankruptcy and hole in the soul. Now, with the legal use of psychedelics, there is a complement of enhancing the opportunity for the spiritual conversion and rebirth experience to happen. Again, the psychedelics are a catalyst, not the cure. The willingness to have the shift in surrendering to something greater than oneself, to a Power Greater than oneself, is a critical component. The psychedelics just make it a little bit easier to get past all the ego defensiveness and blocks to the surrendering process. I have therapeutically prepared and sat with countless people, watching them have a spiritual conversion right before my eyes.

REBIRTH OF THE SOUL

It is like experiencing birth. And it is a rebirth of the soul. There I hear ecstatic utterances of "Oh God, wow, oh God." These utterances may or may not be accompanied by a vision of the light, the voice of God, or the appearance of a form of God or Jesus or Mother Mary with a message. The most prominent message is one of love. Many clients say, "I know I am loved; I know God loves me, I love God, there is so much love helping me right now."

Of course, there is no guarantee that this will happen and some of the most skeptical people I have worked with have had the biggest spiritual conversions. For me, in my work with or without psychedelic medicine, there must be a complement of the spiritual component with the therapeutic work, including family of origin work, as addictions tend to be patterned generationally, along with the fellowship of a loving group that puts the whole package together and makes recovery sustainable. That is why I make the recommendation to work on the Twelve Steps, they are a roadmap for the journey. And to go to meetings and be the energy field of loving and supportive people.

PSYCHEDELICS A HEALING BALM

Psychedelic medicines are not a cure-all. At best, it is a jump-start to the conviction of living a good life. It is the catalyst for working a solid program of recovery and enjoying a new sense of connectedness in relationships. Bill W. demonstrated his determination by continuing to actively work the twelve-step program and apply the principles of AA to his life. Bill W. kept sharing the message of AA of hope and healing with others who were sick and suffering. He made a choice of living sober one day at a time.

Psychedelic medicines can be the healing balm when combined with therapy, rituals of recovery, and the twelve-steps to aid thousands still suffering from a variety of addictions.

Drug rituals also provide meaning and purpose in life, but eventually, it will kill a person or create sickness or disease. Rituals of recovery bring comfort and a sense of belonging. Within that structure of the twelve-steps, there was security and opportunity for experimenting and expanding with parts of ourselves and telling our stories. The experience of sharing one's story reflects how ritual provides a context in which we can grow and discover ourselves.

A POWER GREATER THAN OURSELVES

How do we come into a relationship with powers that are so much bigger than ourselves through rituals? Ritual helps to ground the bigger experiences of life. The ritual helps to give structure to what may be a more chaotic or unstructured experience. It can help make sense of things; it can help to give some security in anchoring the unknown so we can know it. To touch the uncontrollable so that we can have a semblance of order. To open to the ineffable so it becomes something we can taste and even digest. In this way, ritual can provide some security when confronting chaos or things much larger than the self. Rituals can help to handle and incorporate new meaning into life, enhance knowledge, and integrate the deeper wisdom of the self.

LOSS AND ADDICTION

Many people in the devastating clutches of addiction feel lost, and that is one of the main characteristics and descriptions, "I feel so incredibly lost." While working at a recovery center, I met a young man in a group I was facilitating, who was twenty-two years old, clean-cut, full of life, and just had a baby boy. He was struggling to stay in the program and wanted to leave treatment. The entire group was encouraging him to stay. He was just not hearing anything being said. In fact, he had his hands over his ears and refused to listen. His legs were nervously bouncing up and down as if he were already running away.

Despite our best efforts, he left treatment, and within twenty-four hours we were informed he had overdosed and was on life support. His family was devastated. They came to the hospital to say their final goodbyes before pulling the plug. Our hearts were broken. The news ripped through the entire community, and all were in grief and shock. That night after his family took him off life support this young man came to me in a dream. In the dream, he had no ears and no eyes. He said to me with his thoughts, "I did not have the ears to hear or the eyes to see." I spoke with the entire community the next day following the dream visitation and shared how he came with a clear message. The story and the dream have been retold hundreds of times and are still shared today to keep the message going--keep your ears and eyes open!

RAW ARCHETYPES

Jungian Analyst, Robert Johnson, summarizes:

> According to Carl Jung, humanity holds a special role in creation: to contribute to the act of consciousness, and the point of view of morality, in its highest sense. Raw archetypes, like tornadoes, are amoral. A tornado does not care where it touches down or what it destroys; it simply acts as it is meant to act. We have no control over the actions of a tornado. We can, however, come to terms with an archetype--because in a real sense, it is us.

Addictions can be viewed in this way as the archetype of despair and destructiveness. Addiction is like an amoral tornado. It wreaks havoc and pain in the lives it touches. The description refers to people in the worst part of their addiction as being out of control like a tornado and leaving a path of devastation behind them.

CAME TO BELIEVE

Robert Johnson continues the theme of oneness and unity on the inside being restored:

> "Remember, everything comes from one source, and the unity of that oneness can be restored. In Step 2 of the twelve-steps, *Came to believe that a power greater than ourselves could restore us to sanity* clearly is pointing to the one source and how it can be restored."

> Johnson explains:
> A good place to begin our understanding of inner work is with the Nicene Creed, *Credo In Unum Deum*: I believe in one God. Psychologically, this means that there is only one source, one beginning, one unity, out of which all life flows and to which it returns. You cannot get lost because you are already home.

I love this thought so much! Through dreams, rituals, and psychedelics we have an opportunity to find the parts of ourselves and find our way home! To intimately experience a reconnection to the power of our inner-life force from which all life flows and our creative regenerative power brings us home to ourselves.

SPIRITUAL AWAKENING

The process of healing is ongoing as reflected in the twelfth step: *Having had a spiritual awakening as a result of these steps we tried to carry this message to alcoholics, and to practice these principles in all our affairs.* This indicates the whole purpose of the addictive process is to have a spiritual awakening and find our way to ourselves.

David R. Hawkins, MD, PhD, was the Director of the Institute of Spiritual Research, Inc., and Founder of the Path of Devotional Non-duality. A renowned pioneer author, lecturer, and clinician in the field of consciousness writes:

> The 12th Step says the whole purpose of the addictive process was to awaken them and move them from one level of consciousness to another; to go from being asleep and unaware, to being awake, conscious, and aware; to move from being unconscious, irresponsible, and the helpless victim to owning themselves as being spiritually responsible for the happiness and success within their life. This precludes putting the source of happiness outside themselves. Instead, they realize that the source of happiness is the same as the source of life and comes from responsibly owning oneself as a spiritually aware person.

The journey toward happiness and success and owning this as an inside job, not an outer change of circumstance, but an inner shifting and rebirth. As we know, addictions are a progressively deadly disease, and the way to recovery is through becoming more aware and spiritually attuned to life!

Hawkins concludes:

Addictions are progressively fatal diseases, and the only way to recover from them is to become progressively spiritually aware and more conscious. Life itself depends on becoming conscious via major self-confrontation with something that each person's Higher Self has chosen that will force them to grow, because there is no turning back. The only options are to surrender their will to God (that which is Higher than the ego) or go insane and die.

Fortunately for millions of people there is hope and healing, there is a life of living with a conscious contact with a Power Greater than the self.

Hawkins states: "Recovery depends on accepting that there is a step-by-step process for healing, and we can move into the process with a bit of gratitude and maybe even some joy."

INITIATION INTO NEW FEELINGS AND CREATIVITY

For me, working in treatment centers is a deeply rewarding experience. I was fortunate to be working within centers that gave me free rein to create rituals of inner healing, create and facilitate ritual groups, and welcome the work with dreams for inner transformation. Drug and alcohol use are highly ritualized behaviors and, if we are to remove one ritual it was imperative to replace it with another more meaningful ritual. Hopefully, one that was more life-affirming.

This is a story of the unexpected effect that ritual work can have as demonstrated by a practicing attorney in one of my groups, coming to awareness of his deeper feeling of nature. The following story begins to reveal the transformation and movement toward openness that was stimulated by the participation in the *Burning Bowl Ceremony*, (Directions and meditation in Section Ten: Rituals of Healing and Transformation) a ritual of release and cleansing.

At the end of the *Burning Bowl Ceremony* the poem was composed as a creative synthesis. After he did the ceremony, he then received an *Angel Card* with one word on it--*Creativity*. I was leading this ceremony as a part of a group experience.

The attorney shared his story:

> It started out when you handed out the "Angel Cards," and as I remember, the one I got was "creativity." And then I discussed that was one thing I wanted to get back into, poetry and creative writing. Then you said, "Why don't you write a poem about what we did here today?" I sat down and wrote it in one draft and one sitting. I changed one or two words from the whole poem from when I wrote it initially. That came right out. I did it in one sitting, it took me two hours. And that was it, that was the whole thing. And I didn't have any particular feeling when I wrote it. I enjoyed it as I wrote it, it was essentially an intellectual exercise as far as I was concerned. Analyzing my feelings and writing them down, but at an arm's length...In other words, I wasn't actually feeling.

FEELING THROUGH ANALYZING NOT REALLY FEELING

The attorney described the way he analyzed his actions to determine what he was feeling and had rarely felt any of his emotions:

> The way I often find out what I am feeling is I analyze my actions to try to determine what I might be feeling. I rarely directly feel the emotion myself. In other words, I will say, I must be feeling this way because I am acting such-and-such a way. That's my analysis rather than directly feeling the emotion. At this time, I did not feel any emotion. I liked the imagery. It felt good and I was proud of the poem, considering that I hadn't written one in thirty years. I had written a poem and it felt good and I enjoyed doing it.

Burning Bowl

I've been playing the game for many years,
sitting shoulder to shoulder at the bar
With the other players, as the hands are dealt
to us in the smokey gloom, wrapped in glass.
At first I would win a pot or two,
Raking in some smiles, laughter, and fun.
The Dealer grinned and poured me another card.
He was patient because he worked for the house
And he knew the house can never lose.
As the cards got worse I held my hand
Closer to my heart so others could not see,
While I bet pieces of my soul and

The tears of those I loved on losing hands
Other players would win a pot or two
And I would envy their brief bit of joy.
But the game was no longer one of chance,
The odds had flown and there was but one end.
Then I was told, "You cannot win the game
But through God you no longer have to play."
So I brought my losing cards from my heart
And let others see the weak hand I held
Upon which I had wagered and lost so much.
Before the honest flame of their caring hearts
My precious cards twisted into the black
And brittle shapes they had always been.

He continued to share:

It wasn't until I was actually reading the poem out loud
in the group that the emotions surged up—totally caught
me by surprise. I got choked up and cried. It was the first
time I had felt any emotion in a very long time. I had felt
none while I was writing it. It was when I was reading
it out loud and essentially sharing it within the group
that the emotions came up. When I was alone, I mean,
maybe you think it would be the opposite way around,
that I would have the emotion when I was alone and not
have it when I was reading with people. That's not the
way it was at all. It totally caught me by surprise, I hadn't
realized, well, I knew I was describing how I felt, but it
was like looking at a sunset. I wasn't participating in the
feelings at the time I was describing. I don't know how

to explain it. They were my feelings, but I wasn't feeling them. They were filtered or something.

He went on to describe the following about feeling his emotions:

But I actually felt the emotions when I read it in the group. And it caught me completely by surprise and essentially, I think what I felt was, for the first time, I felt the pain of my addiction. And, I didn't realize, I knew that I didn't like it, but I didn't realize how big the pain was. I think that was essentially the emotion I was feeling, the pain part of it. That's what really got me, and of course, I'm not used to feeling feelings so that kind of surprised me, too.

RITUAL WORK IN TREATMENT

In this very intimate story, we begin to see the process of openness and initiation into new life through a group and community experience. Even in his description of his stages, we see the willingness to open to a deeper level and then almost as a surprise, moving into a new life experience within the group.

The rituals helped this man and many others connect with his inner world and deepest feelings of pain and suffering for the first time. He participated in gathering all the fractured parts of himself. During the ceremony and writing of the poem, he began to have a new sense of his inner wholeness, even his holiness. Through the ritual work and creative writing he could see the bigger picture from a new perspective and the gestalt of his entire life. He found his own words, his own story, his own symbols, his own emotions, and images of the card game within himself, which he could share with others in the recovery community through his story and personal poetry writing.

We too can reclaim these parts or our fragmented selves through the journey, using ritual, ceremony, group support, and writing. We can learn to express and experience real joy internally and find a renewed connection with a full range of feelings, including ecstasy and the ecstatic oneness available right now within our inner world. In the sacred space of a caring community, utilizing rituals and ceremony, evoking the non-ordinary state of consciousness, we touch into the experience of the transcendence.

RITUALS, CEREMONY, AND GROUP WORK: ENTERING NON-ORDINARY STATES TOGETHER

Themes keep emerging as we seek to understand and explore more of what it means to enter these transformative states:

1. The unconscious and conscious connecting.

2. The connection to the spiritual realm.

3. The transcendent qualities.

4. The sense of being born with the desire to create ritual.

5. The meaningful patterns of experience.

6. The honoring of community.

7. The marking of rites of passage and initiation, individually and collectively.

Questions for reflection on rituals and recovery:

How can creating rituals help you connect to your inner self and emotions?

....

....

....

....

What have you learned about spiritual bankruptcy and the hole in the soul?

....

....

....

....

What does a Power Greater than yourself mean to you personally?

....

....

....

....

How could you create a ritual to honor your own rite of passage into new life and recovery?

....

....

....

....

How can you use rituals and community support in recovery?

....

....

....

....

How can you creatively become a spiritually aware and conscious person?

....

....

....

....

How can the twelve-steps, transformative rituals, and psychedelic medicine used together, play a role in healing from a sense of separation from yourself and finding your way home?

....

....

....

....

9

Psychotherapy Tools for Triggers and Boundaries

Understanding how to use basic psychotherapy with psychedelics is very important. Our thoughts and feelings are triggers for our actions or reactions and are the core of Cognitive Behavioral Therapy (CBT). We need to have some understanding of these basic skills and tools, which are essential for working on ourselves, or if you are a therapist or facilitator working with your clients who have their own personal triggers. Dreams and psychedelics may reveal areas of healing that these psychotherapeutic skills and tools will help to address. Psychedelic medicine may illuminate worries, fears, and anxieties, and show areas of growth and opportunity for our inner development. We need to know how to do the mental and emotional work of our healing our responses to triggers.

These therapeutic tools offer specific ways to deal directly with personal empowerment and change how we respond when our buttons get pushed. Defusing our responses to triggers is an inside job. The following are ways to help us keep our cool and confidence when we are emotionally triggered. Additionally, we will learn how to process quickly getting through intense situations and manage our own emotional responses with greater ease and control. No one has power over us unless we give it to them. These tools are simple and effective ways to use that dash of time between getting triggered and losing our peace of mind or sanity. These simple and highly effective tools help us hold on to our personal power and stay confident.

KNOWING ABOUT BOUNDARIES

Healthy boundaries are a big part of getting triggered. Most of the time there has been a boundary crossed and the trauma or hurt has been triggered. Understanding and setting healthy boundaries is part of the process of healing and staying empowered. We all get triggered at times, even when we know what is happening. When we do get triggered how do we get unblocked? When you shut down how can you have self-compassion, self-understanding, and self-forgiveness, and work through the trigger and get unblocked? Sometimes we are the ones triggering ourselves with our own negative loop of thinking and feeling. It is not someone doing something to us, or attacking us, we are triggering or attacking ourselves with our own thoughts. We need to know how to navigate our own internal dialogue and narrative with more awareness and confidence. This process will be shared in detail in this chapter.

BEHAVIOR IS AN INSIDE JOB

The working principle is that when we understand ourselves, it is much easier to understand and deal comfortably with others. By mastering our responses to situations or people who trigger us, we become more skilled at building dynamic personal, and caring relationships with those around us. When we realize how we are triggered, we can prepare ourselves internally to respond more appropriately externally.

The better we understand our personal strengths and weaknesses, the more effective we become at altering our responses to uncomfortable situations. But the effect doesn't stop there. When you are comfortable within yourself, you are more conscious of others' comfort levels, and their strengths and weaknesses. Self-knowledge leads to knowing others as well.

THE DASH OF TIME THAT MAKES THE DIFFERENCE.

We are going to use the acrostic, D-A-S-H, because that is how quickly we can become triggered, and it is just that split second of time that gives us a chance so we don't say or do something we regret later. When you begin to feel as though you are getting your buttons pushed, you only have that split second, that dash of time between the trigger and your response. Here is the quickest way to regain power and peace of mind; remember it is the dash that makes the difference. I suggest using a neuro-linguistic programming technique, touch your thumb to your index finger, and with each letter move to the next finger and progressively say each word then move to the next finger:

D: Defuse
A: Analyze
S: Self-Talk
H: Handle it

TOOL: D-ASH: DEFUSE YOURSELF FIRST

When you are triggered, the first person you need to gain control of is yourself. Stop playing the blame or shame game and finger-pointing. Get control of yourself; you cannot control anybody else. You know you have tried to control other people and it didn't work; they never changed, and you only became more upset and lost more power and peace of mind. Stop trying to control them and take control of yourself by taking total responsibility for yourself your emotions and your perceptions of the situation. First you get control of yourself, then you can begin to control the situation.

This is not always easy to do! You want to blame somebody, and you want to make them wrong, you want to feel self-righteous and better than them. Also, you are angry at yourself for letting someone trigger you. How could you be so stupid? How could you be so unprepared and let yourself get out of control? You feel bad about your own triggered responses, and it makes it harder for you to get unblocked mentally and emotionally.

Everyone makes mistakes. Let go of the fear of being out of control. Defuse yourself first. Gain control of yourself.

Prepare yourself positively by what you say to yourself, your own self-talk; your internal dialogue might be something like this,

"This person is really upset right now; I know it is not about me. They are upset about a situation and taking it out on me. I am going to have to take some extra time to find out what is really going on."

Appear calm, self-assured, and centered even if you may not feel that way. Your anxiety can add fuel to the fire and even escalate tension and aggression. Use a modulated, even, flat tone of voice. If you notice your voice sounding tight, higher pitched, or scared, change or modify it. Lower your voice, ask questions, and wait. Really listen to their responses. Help them save face and you will save face too.

TOOL: DA-SH: ANALYZE THE SITUATION

Analyze the situation. Imagine that you are a detective, and you are carefully putting the pieces of a mystery together. Look for missing information, problem-solve, and look at all the symptoms before making a diagnosis. While you are doing this investigation, be respectful toward them and ask for their help.

Remember, this person believes you have what they need it's information or power to do something that you may or may not have. The person may become more agitated while you are in this inquiry process because they may be very fearful or insecure about their position. Because they are feeling this way, they may be throwing complaints or insults at you. Do not become defensive, this is not about you. It is their anxiety about the situation.

You are observing and assessing the situation, asking questions, and even showing empathy for the person while gathering data. Empathize with feeling not with behavior. For example, "You have a right to be upset but it is not okay to swear at me." Show care and empathy. Apologize, even if you are not involved. Maintain eye contact. Use their name. Sometimes people just need to vent.

TOOL: DAS-H: SELF-TALK

The most important conversation you will have all day long is the one you are having with yourself. What is the internal conversation going on in your head? I am referring to your own inner dialogue; what are you saying to yourself? Becoming conscious of your inner dialogue and the perceptions and pictures you are creating in your mind will help you gain control and assess the situation.

Listen to what you are saying to yourself. Listen to the tone, the words, and the feelings behind the words. We are our own worst enemies at times. We are more critical of our self than anyone else could ever be. Use your self-talk in a more encouraging way. You and I have to be our own best cheerleaders. If you are waiting for someone else to tell you that you are doing a good job, you may be waiting a very long time to get the "good job" or "congratulations" stroke from the boss or someone else.

Recognize your inner voice and tune into what you are saying and use it positively to promote your own inner sense of well-being and self-worth. Sometimes you need to just be quiet, tell the negative inner voice to "be still and sit down," or "thank you for sharing," and move on to the back of the bus.

When you learn to have better control of the inner voice you also maintain better control of the impulse to just blurt something out that may be hurtful or damaging. Silence is always golden. There is a whimsical yet wise phrase: "who you are speaks so loudly I can hardly hear what you are saying." Who you are, how you carry yourself, and your ability to hold your tongue, speaks volumes.

Practice having the emotional and mental maturity to hold your tongue and it will serve you and help you to hold on to your power.

TOOL: DAS-H: HANDLE IT AND MOVE ON

Do whatever you can to take care of this person, serve this person, and move on. Do not dwell on the situation and play it over in your mind, make calls or text about it, or tell family and friends about this horrible encounter you had today. When you and I replay this in our minds we experience all the stress over and over. Let it go. Handle it and forget about it.

HOLDING ON TO YOUR POWER WHILE COMMUNICATING

You and I don't see the world as it is, we see it through our own lenses of perceptions that have been influenced by our beliefs, values, social experiences, and how we were raised as children. We see the world through our own our own personal glasses, which influence how we perceive everything.

To hold on to our power and not become triggered, we need to communicate while owning that we are seeing a situation from our own perception. The following "I" statements will help you focus on sharing in a healthy and productive way that will increase your ability to get your needs met and meeting the needs of others.

Begin to describe the situation using these three phrases:

"I See…"
"I Feel…"
"I Would Like…"

WHAT IS A PERSONAL BOUNDARY?

A personal boundary is the limit you set for your personal, emotional, mental, and physical space.

Some people may imagine their boundary as a protective shield or an attractive fence with a gate or door allowing certain people to have access inside. We choose who we let in and how far we let them in emotionally, mentally, and physically. The doorknob of your life is on the inside.

Boudaries help us be aware of honor, and value our unique individual qualities we bring into the workplace. When someone in our life is angry and directs it toward us with harsh words or actions, we can maintain our boundaries and stand up ourselves. No one is ever meant to be a door mat for others. We remember we're the only ones who can set our boundaries; we cannot rely on others to set our boundaries for us. Some people who have a lack of boundaries will not recognize our boundaries. They actually help us define our individuality and separateness. We must communicate our boundaries to those around us in a gentle but firm way. By keeping our hand on the doorknob on the inside we can open and shut the door when needed, to set a boundary that keeps us safe.

Using our "I" statements in communication, we confront the individual about the anger or lack of boundaries and share our feelings and our personal need for this boundary. We also need to determine what we need to do for ourselves if the boundary continues to be violated.

Over time we learn to have more confidence in our feelings because our feelings tell us when our boundaries have been violated. It sometimes may feel like an internal OUCH! In this way we take better care of ourselves. Remember the only person you can control and have power over is you. We can ask that our boundaries be respected but you cannot control what other people will say or do.

SIGNS OF UNHEALTHY BOUNDARIES:

A person…

- who reveals too many intimate details about their lives,

- goes against personal values or their own integrity to please others,

- who is overwhelmed or pre-occupied with another person,

- who is not noticing when someone else displays inappropriate boundaries,

- who is not noticing when someone invades their boundaries,

- who accepts food, gifts, or touch they do not want,

- who touches another person without asking,

- who takes as much as they can take for the sake of getting,

- who gives as much as they can give for the sake of giving,

- who allows others to take as much as they can from them,

- who allows others to direct their life,

- who lets others describe their reality,

- who believes others can anticipate their needs,

- who expects others to fill their needs automatically,

- who falls apart so someone will take care of them,

- who abuses themselves with alcohol, drugs, food, physical abuse, and work abuse.

WAYS OF THINKING, FEELING, AND PERCEIVING THAT CAN CAUSE ME TO BE TRIGGERED

Some perceptions I come to believe are true, can produce internal conflict and upset and cause me to be triggered. These perceptions are uniquely mine, *I created them, I am reacting to them*, and I may be letting them trigger me. My thoughts and feelings are creating my life experience from the inside out. How am I allowing the power of my thoughts and emotions to get me triggered? The examples that follow are ways I may be using the power of my perceptions to cause me to be triggered. These are the areas in my own thinking and feeling I may need to "Re-Do".

Put a checkmark next to the ones that may apply to you so you can become aware of when you need to have a "Re-Do":

☐ **Exaggerated Thinking is a Trigger:**

I may make my problems bigger than they are and magnify the negative and diminish or minimize the good things happening in my work and life.

☐ Blaming is a Trigger:

When I am blaming myself excessively for all that has gone wrong, I am assuming too much responsibility. When I am excessively blaming someone else or others for what is going wrong, I am in conflict with the world, and all the people around me are at fault. When I am blaming, I am giving my power away. It is not until I take 100 percent responsibility that I can maintain power and keep from getting triggered.

☐ Mind Reading is a Trigger:

When I am predicting the future in a negative way or assuming somehow I can read another person's mind and that I know for certain what is going to happen, I am mind reading. Anytime I jump to quick conclusions without checking out the facts and go on to make my own interpretation of the facts, I am mind reading.

☐ Negatively Labeling Yourself or Someone else is a Trigger:

When I call myself a name, like loser or stupid or not good enough, I am labeling, and I will end up with a sense of hopelessness and helplessness for the future. If I am labeling someone else a fool or loser or jerk, I will stop all caring communication in that relationship. Even if I say those mean-spirited names behind their back, at some level they know, and I know that I have said them and it will interfere or block positive communications in the relationship.

☐ All or Nothing Perceptions is a Trigger:

It is either all good or all bad, there is no middle ground. This also includes perfectionism, and if a plan does not turn out perfectly, the whole plan is a failure or no good. It is also called black and white thinking, when really, life is composed of much more gray areas.

☐ Expectations are Thoughts that Produce Triggers:

I tell myself the way things should be, my expectations, and the way I think people should act or behave. When it does not happen, I am resentful and angry. One person put it this way, "Expectations are resentments under construction!"

☐ Dwelling on a Situation is a Trigger:

I am obsessing about the negative side of a situation at the exclusion of seeing any of the positive. I can pick out one scene in my mind that was negative or hurtful and go over it again and again and again. If I am overly sensitive, just one criticism can diminish many positive comments given to me by others.

☐ Discounting is a Trigger:

Accentuating the negative and discounting the positive. I never give myself pat on the back for a job well done. Even if I do a good job, in my mind I may be thinking, "It wasn't really that good. I could have done better." When I am discounting, I never get any strokes, and I will build up resentments and hostility over a period of time. This can be true if I am discounting another as well. They will feel hopeless, as if they will never be able to measure up, no matter how hard they try.

Here is the Antidote and Inner Healing and Turning it Around: Getting Out of Being Triggered

When I am getting my buttons pushed by my own perceptions and ways of thinking here are some quick tips to have a "Re-Do" so I can have enough humility to turn my perceptions around and take ownership and responsibility for my thoughts and feelings.

Put a check mark next to each one you will use, to have an internal and external "Re-Do":

☐ **Balanced thinking:**

I magnify the positive. I see what could work out positively in this situation. I keep the importance and weight of my problems in perspective. I remember that no problem is too heavy when that problem is shared with another. It is vital that I ask for help when I need it. I face my problems one day at a time. I see the best-case scenarios. I remain optimistic while working on my problems. I trust everything I need; I will have.

☐ **I take 100 percent responsibility:**

I neither blame others or myself. I take responsibility for what I need to do to improve my life. I am honest about my own mistakes and shortcomings. I am willing and able to change. I don't take on too much of the responsibility and I don't put the responsibility onto others. I remain in charge of my metaphoric remote control and my channels of thought. I remember the power is in my hands. I am powerful.

☐ When in doubt, check it out:

Never assume anything, (remember, when I make an assumption, I may make an ass of u and me) it makes sense that I can only really know what is going on in my life, not everyone else's.

☐ I speak of myself and others in positive ways:

Give yourself compliments, praise and encourage others, make gratitude and appreciation a part of your daily conversation. Always use kind and gentle words when referring to yourself and others.

☐ Living in shades of gray:

Life is much more a blend of good days and not so good days, and routines and chores, and rarely do things work out perfectly. There are very few absolutes, so I am willing to live with the ambiguity and paradoxes in my life. I let go of the "all or nothing thinking" that is causing stress in my life.

☐ I see the good in myself and others:

When I don't project my expectations onto others, I allow them to be themselves. This also frees me to live without fear of the expectations or projections of others. I am good enough and those around me are good enough. The truth is, you and I are doing our best most of the time, accept this and move on.

☐ **Living in the present moment:**

I only have power to change or "Re-Do" this moment now and possibly make plans to do more changes in the future. I cannot live in the past; the past is over. I cannot live in the future; it has not happened. There is no power in the universe that can change one thing about yesterday; it is done. I need to take today and live it fully with as little regrets and resentment as possible. I remind myself, "Today is the first day of the rest of my life." When I find myself dwelling in the past, I take a mental inventory of lessons learned' mistakes made and move on. If I do not understand or acknowledge my history, I may be destined to repeat it. Once I have learned the lesson, made amends for my mistakes where possible; I need to move on and live in this moment right now.

☐ **I look for the good in every situation:**

Even in the worst situations there can be a ray of sunshine. Dolly Parton once said, "You can't have a rainbow without the rain." When I am faced with obstacles, misunderstandings, and conflicts, I can turn it around inside of me by saying, "I can't wait to see the good that comes out of this!" Believe me, this is an antidote for much of what might otherwise push my buttons. In turning my mind toward what can come out of this positively, I am sending a message to the subconscious mind that I can handle whatever comes my way.

LEARNING SELF-ACCEPTANCE

Part of this process is learning self-acceptance. Accepting myself does not mean that I will never change or have a "Re-Do." In fact, when I accept myself, I am more powerful and capable of making changes. It is about making good choices. When I make a poor choice, I have the ability to have an internal "Re-Do," or if I have made a poor choice in my life and relationships, I can admit it and ask to have a chance to do it again. Arrogance and egotism are defensive-triggered attitudes and behaviors and make it difficult for us to be humble, admit our mistakes, and move forward.

We have to admit our shortcomings in order to progress and move on.

AN INTERNAL RE-DO

We all know the definition of insanity: Doing the same things in the same way expecting different results.

WHEN WE ARE TRIGGERED:

We tend to make more of our mistakes and blunders when we are most depleted. Overeaters Anonymous has a great acronym they use to identify when we are most vulnerable. Under these conditions we will make more mistakes and may need to have more Re-Do's. H-A-L-T is the word which means to stop or halt.

This is what it stands for:

H-Hungry
A-Angry
L-Lonely
T-Tired

When we are aware of any of these, we need to stop! Halt! And take good care of ourselves before we get triggered or we trigger someone else.

REPLACING INNER NEGATIVE SELF-TALK WITH AFFIRMATIONS:

In one of my workshops a working mother had never written or used personal affirmations before. She was asked to write an affirmation and say it out loud to themselves at least fifty times in the morning and fifty times in the evening for thirty days. This is the affirmation and story she shared with the class:

Her Affirmation: *"This is the best day of my life!"*

I would say the affirmation with my three kids in the morning as I was getting them ready for school and driving them to their destinations. One day she reported, "I was running late, I was tired, everything seemed to be going wrong. I flopped down in the car feeling stressed and frustrated and a bit unhappy with myself. My 5-year-old son leaned over the seat and whispered in my ear, "Remember mommy, this is the best day of your life!" My eyes welled up with tears as my son gave me a thousand more good reasons to be happy. I use my affirmations everyday whether I feel like it or not, the kids are getting as much out of it as I am!

Here are a few more of my favorite affirmations. These come from my book *Twelve Powers in You,* in which are written thirty affirmations, one for each day, after each of the Twelve Powers.

I am a tower of strength.

I am wise and use good judgment. I am powerful and full of power.

I understand that at my core I am a good person. I am willing to hear other people's point of view. I am one with all life.

I am alive, I am alert, and I am enthusiastic about my life. I am powerful beyond measure.

So now it is your turn to write your affirmations below. Write the affirmation you will be using for the next thirty days, in the morning and at night:

Affirmation: *"Every day in every way I am getting better and better."*

FOUR STEPS TO SUCCESSFUL AFFIRMATIONS

1. When you create your affirmations make sure that they are written in the present tense and positive. Do not put anything behind the phrase "I AM" that is not positive.

2. Say your affirmations out loud with enthusiasm. Put lots of positive energy, thoughts, feelings, and images in each one as you repeat them aloud.

3. Say your affirmations over and over. It is necessary to self-train a mind that has lived so long in mistakes and bogus beliefs that it needs this constant repetition of positive ideas to create a new you. Repeat them at least fifty times in the morning and fifty times in the evening before you go to bed. Then watch what happens in your life.

Exercise: Write your own personal affirmation:

OUR ATTITUDE MAKES ALL THE DIFFERENCE

Our attitude is one of our greatest assets. Our attitude has power over us whether we realize it or not. Our attitude can create unnecessary barriers to performance or by making simple changes, those barriers to performance can slip away.

William James, a Harvard Psychologist once said:

"By changing the inner attitudes of their minds, they can change the outer aspects of their lives."

Possibly the most important factor in determining our attitudes is paying attention to our thoughts. The thoughts we hold in our mind become our attitude and our lenses of perception. When we change our thoughts we change our feelings and we change our behaviors, and we change our lives. This is how we become resilient!

What thoughts have been holding you back from reaching your goals in life? Challenging My Own Internal Dialogue:

I make the choice every day on how I participate in daily conversations. My own internal dialogue is what I say to myself. My external dialogue is what I say to others. Listening to my internal dialogue is important. One client in a group admittedly never considered listening to her own self-talk. You and I are talking to ourselves all the time and it is good practice to listen to what I am saying to myself and ask myself some helpful and clarifying questions:

What am I saying to myself that has made me so upset or angry?

....

....

....

....

Am I helping myself or hurting myself with what I am telling myself about this person or this situation?

....

....

....

....

Is what I am telling myself true? Do I really have all the facts?

....

....

....

....

Am I really going to take a stand on this situation or am I just making a big deal out of nothing?

....

....

....

....

What can I do or say when I recognize my boundary is being violated? Describe briefly.

....

....

....

....

What can I do to set a healthy boundary and hold on to my power and peace of mind?

....

....

....

....

10

Rituals for Healing and Transformation

Rituals are symbolic ways to celebrate or mark a threshold we cross in our lives individually or as a communal activity when something important happens. We crave fresh rituals that can heal and transform our lives. Rituals give us a depth of knowing ourselves and the meaning and purpose of our existence. Rituals show us how we fit within our own community and our family. These rituals can be adapted and used as part of the pre- and post-integration sessions with the psychedelic medicine journeys. They can also be used as an opening to enter non-ordinary states of consciousness. The rituals will enhance the three inner pathways to help connect with the transcendent dimensions. The end of this chapter includes rituals that can be used for healing and transformation with or without the addition of psychedelic medicines. Guidelines and descriptions of rituals and ceremonies are included.

BIG SUR: ESALEN INSTITUTE EXPERIENCE

I have met some amazing people along the way over the last thirty years, working with rituals and ceremonies, beginning with my first trip to Esalen in 1993. The Esalen Institute is a non-profit American retreat center and intentional community in Big Sur, California, which focuses on humanistic alternative education. The institute played a key role in the Human Potential Movement beginning in the 1960s. I went to study with Stanley Krippner, Professor of Psychology, at Saybrook Institute and

Coauthor David Feinstein of *Personal Mythology and Spiritual Dimensions of Healing*. We created rituals and ceremonies, explored our dreams, and used imagination to enter and deeply understand our own personal mythology and our story. During the experiential workshop, we participated in creating rituals together.

Stan Krippner and David Feinstein define ritual as "a symbolic act that celebrates, worships or commemorates an event or a process in the individuals or the community's life." They described how societies have created rituals to "shape the individual's development, a consequential feat in human engineering. Character traits that served the needs of the clan could be fostered, and the individual's passion and spiritual aspirations could be directed to benefit the community."

CRAVING FRESH EXPERIENCES OF RITUALS

"Rituals may strengthen the rapport with nature," states Feinstein and Krippner. "Rituals delineate the tasks of the individual or community development or establish a connection with aspects of the cosmos that are held to be sacred or divine. A ritual can be centuries old or devised for a contemporary occasion. It might be performed regularly, occasionally, or only once."

They continued, "A ritual can be carried out privately or with others. A private ritual might consist of writing a farewell letter and ceremoniously burying or burning it. Public rituals are typically formed in a prescribed manner and in a certain order, such as graduation, wedding, or funeral. They may be conducted by a family, a small group, or an entire community."

Feinstein and Krippner explained, "Rituals may or may not be accompanied by words, music, or mind-altering techniques such as the whirling dance of Sufi dervishes, Native America peyote ceremonies, or the delirious frenzy of a rock concert." We desire good rituals. They concluded by saying, "Modern people crave fresh rituals, attuned to the times and capable of responding to their higher sensibilities. A growing number of innovative approaches are helping individual and communities rediscover ancient ceremonies and create new rituals."

OUR SOCIETY MYTH DEPRIVED

Stan Krippner was gracious enough to write a review for my very first book published, *Transformative Rituals: Celebrations for Personal Growth*, which at the time I was sending out to different publishers. In his review, he acknowledged how ritual-deprived we are as a culture. "Transformative Rituals is a unique book, its authors have provided their readers with twenty-five exercises in personal transformation that they can use themselves, with their clients, or with groups. Our society is myth deprived, ceremony-deprived, and ritual-deprived. This engaging book tries to redress this imbalance in a way that is both inspirational and practical, both concrete and profound." I am deeply grateful to Dr. Krippner for his teachings and encouragement. Included in this chapter are some of the most popular rituals from my early book.

DANCE OF LIFE EXPERIENCE

One of my favorite shirts I had as a child had a big picture of Snoopy on it. Beneath the picture was the caption "To live is to dance. To dance is to live." Author Ram Dass called one of his books, *The Only Dance There Is*. I have lived the dance in my life. I have lived life to the fullest, pushing boundaries, and assessing the limits. Now I find myself dancing to live, letting the childlike wonder of life dance through me again with all its regenerative qualities. I had studied with Ram Das in Kansas City, Missouri at Unity Temple. I was able to thank him and give him a big hug of appreciation, which he received with joy. Ram Das is an ongoing spiritual presence of healing and transformation for me and my work. One of the key messages I have carried for my entire life journey from him was, "Be here now!" Additionally, "We're all just walking each other home."

DEEPEN OUR INDIVIDUAL LIFE EXPERIENCE

The use of plant medicines and psychedelics with rituals that are transformative has far-reaching implications when done mindfully, carefully, and with therapeutic or facilitating support. For individuals and groups in the community, the implications and applications for the triune pathway are many. Combining all pathways for inner healing and transformation, using dream material, rituals of healing and transformation, and psychedelics, is the powerful triune cord woven for maximum benefit and indelible imprint on the heart and soul.

HEALING CENTERS FOR EVERYONE

There is hope and a vision that one day there will be six thousand health and wellness centers across the United States that offer psychedelic medicines and Psychedelic-Assisted Therapy to healthy people, as well as those struggling with mental health issues and end-of-life stress. The vision is for medical coverage by all insurance carriers including Medicare and Medicaid. It is estimated that psilocybin and MDMA will create ten billion in annual sales, targeting treatment-resistant depression; perhaps replacing drugs like Prozac and Zoloft and other selective serotonin re-uptake inhibitors forever. We have just begun to see the implications and applications for help and a new kind of support for so many sufferings.

The Psychedelic-Assisted Therapy will ideally be open to all people, including people in the general population who want to enter a deeper understanding of themselves. Perhaps mitigating debilitating and consuming life stress that can be crippling for anyone. Helping to turn the tide on burnout and the overwhelming feeling. Possibly offering more options for self-actualization, enhancing creativity, and addressing some of our existential angst.

Sadly, suicide rates are going up at an alarming rate and are now a public health issue. Suicide leaves a lasting impact on families and communities. Suicide is the twelfth leading cause of death in the United States. In 2020, 45,979 Americans died of suicide and there were 1.2 million suicide attempts. The highest rate of suicide is in middle-aged white men. On the average there are 130 suicides per day in the United States. It may be possible to offer a better understanding of the meaning of life, the purpose of our life, and discovering a reason to keep living.

ANXIETY AND DEPRESSION

Implications for dealing with anxiety and depression look promising. General Anxiety Disorder affects approximately 6.8 million adults or 3.1% of the United States Population. Unfortunately, only about 43.2% are even receiving any treatment. Trial studies continue to show a great deal of promise dealing with Post Traumatic Stress Disorder (PTSD), which now affects 7.7 million adults or 3.6% of the entire United States population. Women are five times more likely to be affected than men. Rape is the trigger of PTSD, with 65% of men and 45.9% of women who are raped will reportedly develop the disorder.

Childhood sexual abuse is a strong predictor of the lifetime likelihood of developing PTSD.

OBSESSIVE-COMPULSIVE DISORDER

Implications for Obsessive-Compulsive Disorder (OCD) are also looking hopeful. OCD affects 2.5 million adults or 1.2% of the United States population. Women are three times more likely to be affected than men. The average age of onset is nineteen, with 25% of the cases occurring by age fourteen. One-third of affected adults first experienced symptoms in childhood.

END-OF-LIFE EASE

There is new potential in palliative care to ease some of the end-of-life fears and anxiety that effect 77 percent of those people with a terminal illness. Psychological distress has been associated with greater physical symptoms, severity, suffering, and mortality in cancer patients. Creating better alleviatory care with plant-based medicines, psychedelics, rituals, and dreamwork can be enormously supportive. Counseling with a therapist or facilitator will help to make this end-of-life transition so much easier.

RELATIONSHIP COUNSELING

Couples Counseling would take a great leap forward with the possibility of coming together and then going beyond ego defenses to really connect and bond with one another. The plant medicines, psychedelics, and MDMA have this capability. The support of a relationship therapist or facilitator gives the couple new tools for communication and resolving conflicts. MDMA has been shown to be particularly beneficial for relationship building and healing as it floods the brain with serotonin and allows for a deeper loving connection.

RECOVERY AND TREATMENT CENTERS

The implications and applications for recovery centers are incredibly promising, with new options available for treatment. Almost twenty-one million Americans have at least one addiction, yet only 10% ever receive treatment. Drug overdoses have tripled over the last twenty years, in part because of the Opioid crisis. About 130

Americans die every day from an opioid overdose. Approximately 2.1 million Americans have an Opioid use disorder.

Combining the rituals of a twelve-Step program, sponsorship, therapy, and plant medicines is the best combination for launching a new life-sustaining path forward and addressing our addiction epidemic in the U.S. Alcohol and drug addiction costs the United States economy over $600 billion every year. Additionally, about 20% of Americans who have depression or anxiety also have a substance use disorder.

Recovery for some is dissolving the defense mechanisms and overcoming the denial. Psychedelics can help in breaking down these interior walls and touch into the experience of a power greater than themselves. To get past the default mode and their personal ego. To have a compelling experience with the Inner Healer which can begin to restore sanity. Enhancing access through psychedelic medicines could open the opportunity for achievable spiritual breakthroughs and mystical illumination.

GLOBAL COMMUNITY AND OUR ENVIRONMENT

The implications and applications for the triune pathway to our global community are so relevant in our world today. With our ozone layer fading, our topsoil eroding, and species of animals becoming extinct, we need to honor the earth and all creation through rituals and honoring our Mother Earth and all life forms.

We also see a return of the beautiful earth-honoring rituals and a deeper respect and reverence for Gaia our Mother Earth. We hold the vision of celebrations for the earth and push to recycle and reforestation taking place. But we need to do more and do it consistently. Psychedelic medicines can reconnect us to nature in more intimate and loving ways. Also, there are many organizations working across the United States and globally toward the decriminalization of nature for all plant-based medicines, so that all of nature is legal and accessible for personal pleasure, personal use, for us all to enjoy.

ENDING WAR AS A GLOBAL RITUAL

We are still seeing war as a needed global ritual. War does not have to be a rite of passage to peace. There are other ways. We must confront and change the need or desire to send people off to military campaigns to come back to their tribe and be declared full-grown people. There are better ways to initiate our youth. That would be my wish for some of the future aspects of positive rituals. I pray that we find other rituals that bring life and construction rather than death and destruction. We are finally seeing the fragility of our planet and its inhabitants on our little spaceship earth, which is our only round little schoolhouse with no sides to it. As Buck Minster Fuller and many others have said, "we all live here together, one planet, one whole earth. We cannot use nuclear war and nuclear threats to resolve international conflicts."

Stan Grof writes in *The Cosmic Game:*

"The current global crisis is of a psycho-spiritual nature. It is therefore hard to imagine that it could be resolved without a radical inner transformation of humanity and its rise to a higher level of emotional maturity and spiritual awareness."

A message that has been repeated over and over again by exploring the triune pathways for healing and transformation. We are not hopeless. There is hope, there is always hope. The triune pathways can open us to our deeper levels of existence and inspire us internally to be called to action. We can be inspired to resolve our global crisis. With our unitive consciousness, we can help to accelerate our conscious evolution of the species, and improve our chances for survival, and have a peaceful coexistence.

WORSHIP SERVICES

There are implications and applications for clergy and the church and a new experience of worship within a community of people. These non-ordinary states of consciousness reveal a tremendous amount about who we are, what we believe, and what is of value. Our state of sacred consciousness can reflect like a mirror of our spiritual life and inner world.

Historically, psychedelics have been used for worship in ancient cultures for thousands of years. The past traditions of the shamans continue in many indigenous cultures. The Native Americans are using peyote in their religious ceremonies. In our Western society, many churches are empty, and so many of the people are spiritually bereft. What would it look like to have a shared mystical experience using entheogens as a Eucharist? To ingest the "Flesh of the Gods," as the mushrooms are sometimes referred to in a more contemporary way.

Transformative rituals, meditation, prayers, fasting, dancing, labyrinth walking, and sacred ceremonies are all a part of creating a non-ordinary state that is life enriching and powerful. Each bring their own impact--opening the community to non-ordinary states. Could we also consider designing ways to also include psychedelics into worship?

In a few spiritual communities in the United States, they are using the entheogen as the sacrament. This mystical path is being explored to enhance community and bring worship to life. The revelation of the Spirit can happen in a dynamic way with all sharing the power and experience of entering the transcendent realms. We can bring a little more heaven to earth and truly touch the transcendent together. We are just seeing how this may evolve in the west.

COUNCIL ON SPIRITUAL PRACTICES (CSP)

The Council of Spiritual Practices is a nonprofit organization established by Bob Jesse in 1993 and "dedicated to making direct experience of the sacred more available to more people." CSP helped organize and fund the first experiments in psychedelic research at Johns Hopkins; CSP also supported the suit that resulted in the 2006 Supreme Court decision recognizing Ayahuasca as a sacrament in the UDV Church. In 1995, CSP developed and published the *Code of Ethics for Spiritual Guides,* that over the years many underground psychedelic guides have adopted. Please refer to csp.org.

FAMILY RITUALS AND CEREMONIES
AND RITES OF PASSAGE

Our families can create and develop meaningful rituals that enhance the love and closeness within a family. Rituals can help bring closure and aid in the handling of death, divorce, and transitions. Like moving to a new home that occurs in every family, rituals can be created to honor endings and beginnings. Creating more conscious and meaningful rituals develops bonds and rites of passage within the family environment. Imber-Black, Roberts, and Whiting feel that "family ceremonies and traditions can be helpful in maintaining stability and minimizing psychological stress within families."

When simple family rituals are maintained, like eating dinner together, it can bring stability to a family. Particularly if the family is going through any family changes: illness, death, divorce, economic stress, or addictions. The daily morning rituals, nighttime rituals, prayer times, after-school rituals, movie time rituals, game/ sports rituals, reading rituals, all help hold the family together.

Cultural rituals and rites of passage and ceremony can enhance the sense of history and lineage and give strength to the roots of the family. To grow, children need roots and wings. The roots to anchor them in their family heritage, and wings to fly and make their dreams come true.

DIFFERENCES BETWEEN RITUAL EXPERIENCES AND PSYCHEDELIC EXPERIENCES

The experience of ritual is a bit different from the psychedelic medicine journey. Both can bring in a new sense of aliveness. The rituals can be more extroverted and an outer experience. One friend described her ritual experience as:

> Very much an energizing aliveness that I would experience in rituals. Dance comes in quite a bit in rituals as I've experienced it. We danced around the house. The

physical experience feeling very alive. Feeling a lot of physical energy in those rituals. Feeling a lot of sound energy, making a lot of sound. Really using all the senses involved, sound and smell, and taste, and clothing, so touch, you know the feeling on my skin, all those things. Contact with other people.

Breathing together. So, the physical, all the senses would be very alive, very alive.

PSYCHEDELICS AND THE FUTURE OF HUMANITY

Stan Grof spoke at the conference on Psychedelic Science in 2017 and shared an overview of what he had observed as the results of using psychedelics responsibly. The list was impressive, including the healing of emotional, psychosomatic, and interpersonal problems.

These were the highlights from the list of his observations of the benefits of the non-ordinary states. Notice how many connect with the larger sense of positive community connections being enhanced:

- Significant decrease in aggression and emergence of compassion.

- Development of racial, sexual, political, and religious tolerance.

- Inner peace, improved self-image, self-acceptance.

- Increased creativity, self-realization, self-actualization.

- Reduction of irrational drives and ambitions.

- Competitiveness replaced by synergy, cooperation wu wei.

- Shift of focus from the past and future to the present moment.

- Increase of zest, joi devivre, love of life, appreciation of beauty.

- Enjoying everyday activities, people, nature, music, food, love making.

- Love of nature and emergence of great ecological sensitivity.

- Sense of belonging to humanity and planetary citizenship.

- What Buckminster Fuller called "Spaceship Earth" from the experiences of the first astronauts looking back on the earth.

- Emergence of the spirituality of universal, non-denominational, non-sectarian, all-encompassing, all-inclusive, and mystical nature.

TRANSFORMATIVE RITUALS AND CEREMONIES

Spiritual Naming Ceremony:

During the Women's Wisdom Weekend retreats, we shared a naming ceremony by allowing a new name to come to us. This is a name we get from our own inner world, naming our own inner experience and our opening to the life of the spirit and our unique sacred nature. This is an initiation into the wisdom we are allowing to come to us. We then created a ritual of empowering ourselves with our new name. One of the experiences I had with this ritual was humorous and touching. I was the organizer and facilitator of the retreat, and it was a large responsibility with many detailed tasks.

When I was leading the group in the opening meditation for the spiritual naming, a quiet voice spoke to me within and said my spiritual name was Gay *Yin*. I laughed inwardly because I really needed a lot more *Yin* energy in my life at that time. I received a truly clear message of needing more time to allow and let myself relax, calm myself, meditate, and be, allowing more of the *Yin* energy to flow through me and balance with my Yang energy.

This Spiritual Naming ritual works well as an introductory group experience. It is especially effective if the therapist or facilitator is working from a transpersonal psychological perspective. The concept of spiritual names is not specific to one belief. Perhaps some discussion between working with the spiritual realm and religious beliefs. The understanding of the transpersonal or spiritual perspective transcends the creeds and dogmas of specific religions.

Spiritual Naming Meditation:

Close your eyes and let yourself breathe and relax. Reflect for a time on where your name came from. Did it come from your parents? How do you feel about your name? Does it fit you? Meditate for a few minutes on the question, "Who am I?" What comes forth in your mind as you ask this question? Is it a name? A quality? An affirmation of your own uniqueness? It is a descriptive word with the same letter as your first name, such as "Powerful Pat."

Use this name as your first name or your middle name. Sometimes a spiritual teacher gives you a name. Giving a spiritual name has been a long-standing tradition in many cultures: African, Asian, Native American, and Hebrew. Jacob became Israel after he wrestled with the angel. Jesus gave Simon his name––Peter the Rock. Saul became Paul after his conversion experience, which started on the road to Damascus. Richard Alpert became Ram Das after receiving his spiritual name from his guru and teacher. Oprah Winfrey was named Orpah on her birth certificate after the biblical figure in the Book of Ruth.

Let a spiritual name come to you; think of the qualities you would like to express through this name. (Pause for a time of silence.)

After a few minutes, conclude the meditation and have the group write and share their spiritual name. Ask them to share briefly with the group the meaning of their spiritual names. Give them some time to conclude the sharing, then ask people to stand in small circles, joining hands.

Energizing Healing Circles:

1. Form a group in a circle of five to seven people, each person takes a turn in the middle of the circle.

2. Hold hands, left hand palm up, right hand palm down, to open the energy flow. Stay silent for a few minutes.

3. One person gets in the middle of the circle. Outside people each rub hands together for a few times.

4. Cup hands over the person in the middle of the circle, bringing in the energy of the sky. Visualize raindrops sprinkling all around them. The person in the middle should take energy into every area of their body, especially any areas that need healing.

5. Now outside people take the energy from the earth, sweeping upward with their hands, beginning at the person's feet. Repeat the person's spiritual name or healing word they have chosen over and over as energy is transferred up their entire body. Outside people shake hands off when they are finished. Let the person in the middle have time to savor the energy for a moment before re-entering the outer circle. Repeat the process with each person.

The Burning Bowl Ceremony:

Give each person a piece of paper and something to write with. Encourage them to complete a brief synopsis of what they want to cleanse or release from their lives. Have metal bowl or container for burning in safely.

Burning Bowl Meditation:

The Burning Bowl Ceremony is a symbolic way to cleanse our lives, to let go of the mistakes and failures of the past, and to move on. The fire in the Burning Bowl is a symbol of transformation. The fire takes the paper and changes it from one form to another. Likewise, in our lives we take these blocks, fears, old hurts, and mistakes and burn them. This releases our personal power, freeing it up to work in our lives in a more constructive way. We realize it takes a lot of energy to keep mistakes and fears hidden. Now is the time to let them go. Now is the time to take that energy and choose to use it in a way that is conscious and life-enhancing. Begin to allow some of the things you want to let go in your life to come to your mind.

As we approach the end of this meditation, we will have the opportunity to write some of these things down on our paper. Let them come to you in an effortless way now, not trying to force or make them up. Just let them come to you, and as they do, slowly open your eyes and write them on the paper. You may want to start your writing with "I am free from…" Take some time and write, then close your eyes again and let another thought come to you and write it down. Take as much time as you need. Today is a new and fresh day. Today we are new people, meeting life in a new way.

After meditation let people come up one at a time or form a line depending on the size of the group. Let each person ignite their papers with a lighter, or Sterno, or in an outdoor campfire if outside.

In large groups in a spiritual community, we invite over one thousand people each year to join the spiritual community in the New Year's Eve Burning Bowl Ceremony, releasing the old year and welcoming the new.

Life Symbol Ceremony:
To gain more insight into ourselves and each other, we shared in creating a Life Symbol Ritual. During this creative ritual, we allowed a symbol that represented our life to come to us and be formed by using a long thin piece of wire. Symbol making is an ancient means of accessing an unconscious and yet deeply meaningful part of ourselves.

Give each person a two-foot piece of wire or colorful pipe cleaners. As they hold the wire in their hands, ask them to think about their lives. What does their life mean to them? How do they feel about their lives in this moment now?

Life Symbol Meditation:

Each of our lives are important. Each of us is a unique, special individual. Each of us has a special gift that we are to give the world—a gift that only we can give.

Think of your life and what it means. What is going on? What do you desire. What do you hope for? Think about the joy and sorrow you have experienced. You are a significant person, a divinity, a richness, a life energy. You are a living soul. From the creation of the universe, through eons of evolution, you have appeared in this place. You have your own memories, loves, and fears. You have your own way of seeing and feeling things. You have the strength of decisions and assent. You have a center of existence. You cannot be anyone other than yourself.

So, let us discover something more of what it means to be yourself. Take the wire in your hands. Relax, let your creative energies surface—don't worry about being artistic. There is no right or wrong way to do this—just your way. Work the wire into a form, a symbol, a shape which represents you and your life. Let the shape come to you from within. Just quietly reflect and let it come. Let the wire move in your hands into a symbol of your life. It can be a sun, an arrow, a peace symbol—anything that represents you and your life. Please work in the silence so we can all listen to our inner voices.

When everyone has finished, ask people to introduce themselves and share their symbol and what it means to them. If the group is larger, break them up into mini groups of five to seven people so everyone has a chance to share that wants to. When the larger group comes together have a few select people share with the larger group.

White Stone Ceremony:

During the White Stone Ceremony, each person was given a small slab of marble or one square tile to do the White Stone Ceremony. Each person was asked to contemplate their own fresh start, a new beginning, and clean slate, having a new opportunity to create our life experience anew at any time. Beginning from within and letting come forth a new name written on the stone taken from the Bible scripture in Revelation 2:17 and they will be given a white stone and in it a new name written.

> "Whoever has ears, let them hear what the Spirit says to the churches. To the one who is victorious, I will give some of the hidden manna. I will also give that person a white stone with a new name written on it, known only to the one that receives it."

–Revelation 2:17 The New International Version (NIV)

White Stone Ceremony Meditation:

To those that overcame, who were victorious, who moved forward with faith, a new name was given. Today we will meditate on our new name, for each of us have overcome adversity. We have freed ourselves to live more fully, conscious of Spirit, Inner Healer, in every aspect of our lives. Our creative life forces our hidden manna.

The custom in the ancient days, when a prisoner was released from prison or bondage, was to give that person a white stone to show they were free. Feel the smooth stone in your hand and know that it represents release from old ways of thinking—limiting ways of expressing your creative life force your inner healing intelligence. Say to yourself, "I am free, I have a clean slate, I can choose any moment to begin again. This is a new beginning, a new day, a new opportunity."

Begin to reflect on a new name. Let it come to you easily without trying to make it happen. Let a name come to you that marks your new beginning. Feel the stone in your hand. Hear it beckon to you. What will your life be called? Is it a name? Is it a tile? Is it a quality? A new state of being? You may want to start with the words, "I am" and then express what you want to see happen in your life. What will be written on your stone? (Period of silence.)

If it is appropriate to the setting, group sharing might follow the time of reflection and writing to build bridges between one's inner world and relationships with family, friends, and community. No one must share if they want to keep it private. Because of the highly personal nature of each revelation, the utmost respect needs to be shown for each person's sharing.

Phoenix Rising Meditation: Meditation for Transcendence:
See in your mind's eye, the phoenix as it is rising out of the flames, the symbol of rebirth. The phoenix comes from Egyptian mythology. The miraculous bird was the embodiment of the Sun God. According to legend, the bird lived five-hundred years, then sacrificed itself to burn on a pyre. But the bird did not die, it rose in youthful freshness to live again. The phoenix is often used as a symbol of immortality.

Let this bird remind you now of your winged, transcendent self—the part of you that is immortal. You, as the phoenix, are a miraculous being. You as the phoenix, can rise from the ashes to the freedom and freshness of new life.

It is from the powerful presence of your transcendent self that is within that you are transformed. You are creation clothed in flesh. All freedom begins with your awareness and conscious connection to the transcendent within you. The thoughts held in your mind at this moment are providing that connection. (Pause.)

In every one of us, there can be thoughts and feelings that keep us from experiencing freedom and our conscious contact with inner wisdom. Let come to your mind some of what you may want or need to let go of so that you can rise out of these ashes. Some of these ashes of insecurity, anger, guilt, perfectionism, worry, procrastination, envy, impatience, blame, indecision, or jealousy. These are normal to feel on occasion, but any of them in excess can begin to limit and consume life energies. In your thoughts, briefly reflect on what behaviors you would like to turn to ash and rise from, renewed. (Pause)

Affirm in your own mind, "My winged transcendent self, over-comes even the most difficult or long-term problems. (Repeat this slowly again.) "I rise as the Phoenix out of the ashes to new freedom."

Now, let come to your mind in the next moments of silence a word or two that are symbols of your freedom. Let come to your mind a word or two that symbolize your transformation. Let words such as acceptance, generosity, faith, humility, trust, forgiveness, love, patience, praise, honesty, action, inner reliance, laughter, life, order, strength, truth, and spiritual awakening come to your mind. Be guided to the word or words that best describe the qualities you would like to express. Let the words come to you in the next moments of silence.

(Pause)

Remember the words, keep them in your mind, and say them to yourself now, several times. (Pause)

Each day is another opportunity to know your freedom, to rise again. "And still I rise." Say this silently to yourself or out loud if you wish, "And still I rise." "And still I rise." "And still I rise." Now take a moment to feel that power moving through you from the tips of your toes to the top of your head. Know when you return from this meditation the transformation will have begun in you.

Write what comes to you after this meditation. If you are in a group, each can share their own inner healing and connection with the transcendent self within.

Appreciation Celebration:

Have people sit in the circle. Ask for one person at a time to come to the center, sit or stand with their eyes open or closed—whatever makes them comfortable. Ask people to tell them something positive: a blessing, praise, appreciation or even a positive word. The person receiving the positive words should say nothing and really take in what is being said. Each person takes a turn in the center. The people in the circle sharing the appreciation are not to be called on or required to speak in order. Anyone can talk, but no one must talk. Encourage people to make comments as individualized as possible. Make sure no one is making any qualified statements, such as, "You have made a lot of progress, but you still need to overcome your fear." The comments or appreciation should be totally positive and supportive.

Letter To and From Higher Power:

The letter to Higher Power can help us seek a new direction by tapping into the transcendent dimension of our inner power from which we can always find the answers to our questions and the strength to carry out our plans. This is a nice closing ritual and can be put in an envelope, sealed, addressed, and mailed back to the participant at a later time if possible.

A letter from Higher Power is an effective way to establish an inner dialogue. The letter can be a dialogue or prayer in the truest sense, allowing us to open ourselves to a deeper contact with our Divine Self. True communion can emerge from the consciousness of the Inner Healer within us, speaking to us intuitively. Since turning within and letting intuition or the inner voice of wisdom speak or write through us may seem quite different, ask them to start by writing their own name.

> Dear_____. Then just sit quietly and listen and let the words come from within and trust the letter and words will come once we open ourselves to the flow of the infinite creative process.

These letters can be highly personal, so sometimes it is better to seal them in an envelope and just mail them back to the person at a designated time on a later date. If the desire to share individual letters is appropriate, let the group be the sacred witness to the internal communication.

Community Love Picture Ritual:
People often have a challenging time expressing their feelings verbally. This can be especially true in a group setting. The Love Picture is a way to open communication through artistic expression on paper. It is a group experience, emphasizing, accepting, and giving group support and love.

Needed: One long roll of paper rolled out on a table or floor. Art supplies: crayons, colored pencils, chalk, old magazines, glue, tape, string, yarn, leaves that have fallen from the trees, tape, scissors, aluminum foil, and colored paper. We want people to express themselves artistically on paper by using art supplies.

To get people thinking, questions can be posed to the group such as:

How do I feel about myself in this group? How do I feel about others in the group?

How can I best use the support of others as I grow and change? What does it feel like for me to ask for help?

How would I describe the experiences of love, support, or help?

Continue by telling the group:

"We will communicate by drawing or writing on the paper. It is a fun way to better understand ourselves and each other. You can write or draw whatever you want. This whole experience will be done in silence. There will be no verbal exchanges. Put something on the paper that describes your feelings about yourself and where you are in the group. As you see others write or draw things, you can communicate with them. For instance, someone may draw a wall, you think, to represent themselves. You might draw a rose climbing up the wall as your message or feeling about them or yourself overcoming the wall.

Nonverbal communication is okay—such as a smile, nod, shake of the head, or pointing. The Love Picture should be completed in silence so that all the group's energy will go toward expressing their feelings on the paper. In closing ask people to gather around the Love Picture and share their meaning of their drawings and what the experience was like for them. You can ask questions such as, "How did you feel when someone drew the rose climbing up your wall?"

Inner Mapping:
Supplies needed: Scissors, glue, construction paper, markers, and old magazines or printed pictures. This ritual is an individual experience of reflecting briefly on an aspect of their life they wish to focus on for growth, guidance, and understanding. Cutting out words and pictures to represent that area of growth and paste them on paper as a collage of thoughts, feelings, and desires to create a visual Inner Map, leading us deeper into our hearts and souls—to our very essence.

Through designing and sharing the Inner Map, we creatively participate in inviting new images, metaphors, and symbols to guide us in our evolution. The word metaphor comes from the Greek and means "to carry over." This experience, which taps into our inner realm of wisdom and guidance, is not the same as "Treasure Mapping," which is often used by those seeking material gain. Inner Mapping brings forth spiritual and mental growth. The images come like dreams to transform our lives and bring in renewed vitality. These images and symbols become like little stepping stones to our inner world, guiding our lives with powerful pictures that can tell an entire story about our experiences. Inner Mapping helps us to understand our sacred story by providing guiding images and metaphors for the journey.

Candle Lighting Ceremonies:

The use of fire was critical to human evolution. By learning to develop and control it, humans were able to cook, make heat and light, construct tools and clay pots, and clear land for farming. Civilizations developed based on the ability to smelt and form metals. Fire has always been worshipped by humans for its beneficial uses when controlled and its awesome power in nature. It has been central to many religions--symbolic of the Divine, home and family, purification, immortality, and renewal. Perhaps because it is so deeply ingrained in our history and evolution, the dancing flames of a fire appear mystical and sacred. Candle lighting ceremonies, which use the power of fire, can be moving, powerful experiences to commemorate special occasions such as a graduation, holiday, or end of a retreat.

Different Variations on the Candle Lighting Ritual:

A candle lighting ceremony can be a meaningful culmination to a graduation by having students light their candles as they walk up on the stage to receive their diplomas. As they light their candles they complete the statement, "I light this candle in honor of...." or "I light this candle as a symbol of..." When I received my master's degree from the Center for Humanistic Studies, every student had a chance to reflect for one minute on the graduation experience and light their candle. This was a nice touch to the graduation ceremony because it allowed for students to share their rite of passage through stories in one phase of their mutual growth and struggles in completing their degree.

Opening Candle Lighting for Retreat Introduction:

This ceremony is designed to help people get to know each other in a group or retreat setting. Have people gather into groups of four or five and give everyone a candle. Begin the ritual with an opening poem or invocation appropriate for the group and this occasion. Play soft background music. Ask people to take their lit candle around the room, silently walking and stopping occasionally to make eye contact with others. Have them reflect for a moment on the spark, inner light, and radiance they see in the eyes of each person. If they choose, they can exchange their candles with each other. After about ten minutes, have everyone return to their small groups and share the feelings and thoughts that came to them as they participated in this ritual.

End of Retreat Candle Lighting:

As I was leading Women's Wisdom Weekends and Spirit Healer Retreats, we would share in a twelve-hour silence. The silence closes with the Candle Lighting Ceremony. Each person lights their candle in front of the entire group, completing the statement, "I light this candle in honor of..." or "I light this candle as a symbol of..." Participants find this is a powerful release of energy collected in the rite of silence.

Burning candles become a visual symbol of the flame of life that illuminates our hearts and heals us at our innermost level.

Family Candle Lighting Ceremony:

This activity can take place in a family gathering, community, church, or synagogue setting. Create a pretend campfire, fill a metal tub with sand, and insert a candle for each member of the family or person participating. As the candles are lit, each person can share a thought on, "What my family means to me." They complete statements such as: "My family is special because…" or "I like being in my family because…" After everyone shares their special thoughts, snuggle up around the campfire of candles, sing songs, and tell stories.

Holiday Candle Lighting Ceremony:
Kwanzaa, Christmas, Hanukkah, Buddhism, Hinduism, and many other traditions and spiritual communities celebrate by lighting candles as part of their celebrations. One unique way this can be done is to include a spiritual message, which is to prep-wrap around the base of each candle with a small rubber band, attaching a verse or affirmation from the tradition or teaching. People are instructed to remove their verse before they come up to the front and light their candle from a larger candle, representing the great light in which we are all a part of the spark of Divinity. Large trays are filled with salt and each candle placed in the trays stands up next to all the others, forming a bright radiance and glow of candlelight. Songs can be sung, prayers can be shared, affirmations repeated together.

Suggested Twelve Powers in You meditation:
Each line can be shared and then repeated in unison with a pause and time for reflection following each one.

> Before Spirit's holy altar within me,
> I light my candle of Faith.
> Before Spirit's holy altar within me,
> I light my candle of Strength.
> Before Spirit's holy altar within me,

I light my candle of Wisdom.
Before Spirit's holy altar within me,
I light my candle of Love.
Before Spirit's holy altar within me,
I light my candle of Power.
Before Spirit's holy altar within me,
I light my candle of Imagination.
Before Spirit's holy altar within me,
I light my candle of Understanding.
Before Spirit's holy altar within me,
I light my candle of Willingness.
Before Spirit's holy altar within me,
I light my candle of Divine Order.
Before Spirit's holy altar within me,
I light my candle of Enthusiasm.
Before Spirit's holy altar within me,
I light my candle of Release.
Before Spirit's holy altar within me,
I light my candle of Life.

You have placed your candle in a bed of salt. There it is shining and adding its brightness to the illumination of the world. The bed of salt represents the earth and all creation, for we are indeed the salt of the earth and one with the creative process. Here at the altar of your own heart you lit your candle of prayer and reflection. This light represents a new birth of Spirit within you. Walk lovingly, respecting all life, using wisely the powers you have been given. Walk serenely in the light of love.

World Celebration Ceremony

The world is a beautiful patchwork quilt of diverse cultures held together by the common threads of belief and humanity. Yet sometimes the differences that make our world so interesting are causes for strife and social unrest. The world celebration ceremony is a symbolic means of honoring and celebrating the diversity of cultures and beliefs so that we can work together and live together in peace.

The ritual: Gather as a family or group of people to celebrate diversity and the oneness of humanity. Readings and candle lighting can be done by designating participants before the ceremony.

Opening: May the leaders of all countries and the people of all races be guided to understand that we are all physically and spiritually one; Physically one because we are descendants of common parents, the primordial father and mother; Spiritually one because we are the immortal children of one spirit, eternally linked in the family of humanity.

First reading and candle lighting:

O Cosmic light, in this silence, takes away the darkness of age. May we realize that thy light illumines all paths. We honor those who walk the path of Hinduism. (Light the first candle.)

We, two, feel the great Om of spirit as it invites us to cultivate peace in our minds, in our hearts, and in our world. (Observe silence.)

Second reading and candle lighting:

Blessed by the power of the Spirit's illumination we understand the truth of those following the teachings of Buddha in their quest for peace; "There is no greater happiness than peace." We honor brothers and sisters who follow the path of Buddha. (Light the second candle.)

In thy blessed light, I shall remain awake forever.
(Observe silence.)

Third reading and candle lighting:

The Cosmic Light illumines the minds and hearts of those who follow Tao. There is a thing inherent and natural that existed before heaven and earth. It stands alone and never changes. It pervades everywhere and never becomes exhausted. I do not know its name. I call it Tao and name it supreme. Its nature is peace, its essence is light. We honor those who follow the Tao (Light the third candle.)

The Tao follows its intrinsic nature, peace, and light. (Observe silence.)

Fourth reading and candle lighting:

I am beholding the Light through the eyes of all. I am working through the hands of all. I am walking through all feet. The followers of the prophet, Mohammad, in their awareness of the Great Allah from the book, The Koran, echo these words; "I will guide you from the darkness of war to the light of peace."

We honor those who walk the path of Mohammed.
(Light the 4th candle.)
"And Allah calleth you into the abode of peace and guideth ye in the straight way."
(Observe silence.)

Firth reading and candle lighting:
Again, the light of spirit manifests as wisdom behind human reasoning. We see the deeper significance of the Judaic covenant with Isaiah; "And my people shall dwell in a peaceable habitation and in quiet resting places." We honor those who walk the path of Judaism. (Light the 5th candle.)

We make this scripture true as we transform fear, resentment, and greed into love, understanding and sharing in God's holy light. (Observe silence.)

Sixth reading and candle lighting:
I will follow the shepherd of peace, guided by the star of wisdom to the birth of Christ consciousness; The Light of love illuminates all who walk the path of Christianity. I honor those who walk the path of Jesus. (Light the 6th candle.)

"Blessed are the peacemakers for they shall be called the children of God."

(Observe silence.)

Seventh reading and candle lighting:

"Come sit with me and let us smoke the pipe of peace and understanding. Let us touch. Let us, each to the other, be a Gift as is the Buffalo. Let us be meat to nourish each other that we all may grow."

Our Native American brothers and sisters called it the Sun Dance. They explained it this way; "This mound of earth is the sacred mountain. These four stakes around the mound are your first four chiefs: One is north, one is south, one is east, and one is west. This fifth stick in the center of the mound is the Peace Chief. This Chief is the one all the rest danced to."

We honor those who follow the spirit of the Peace Chief. (Light the 7th candle.)

Our own vision quest is the peace, peace, peace. (Observe silence.)

CONCLUSION

I am the All, from which All proceedeth. With thy mind and understanding fixed firmly upon me, thou shalt come to me. By whatever path you seek me you will find me. We respect and recognize our sisters and brothers who walk the non-sectarian path, and who view the Absolute from a non-parochial perspective. True spirit lies beyond the realm of the visible. In each, there is a spark able to kindle new fires of peace and human progress. When enough fires are burning, they will create a new dawn of spiritual understanding. The flame of great peace will be formed. Humankind will advance to a higher level of civilization.

Responsive affirmation

(Read then repeat together)
I am a spark of the infinite.
I am the darkness and the light.
The Spirit of Peace directs my thoughts and my actions.
The ceremony could be concluded with a circle dance a
song or simply dismiss in the silence.
(The World Celebration ceremony was created by
Sandra Weisner and adapted for use here.)

CLOSING THOUGHTS ON THE
PARADOXES OF THE JOURNEY

- Letting go of yourself
  to find yourself.

- Going into the darkness
  to find the light.

- Being alone only to find
  you are never alone and
  always connected.

- To go a-way to find
  there is no-a-way.

- Going deeply within oneself
  to find a way out of oneself.

- To use a psychedelic drug to
  get off an addictive drug.

- To be blindfolded with an
  eye mask to really see.

- To leave oneself completely
  to find oneself complete.

- To be quiet in order to
  hear silence and know,
  beyond knowing.

- To enter fears of the unknown
  to find that you know
  more than you could ever

realize about everything except maybe yourself.

- To get to the end of everything you know and realize there is volumes more to still explore and the library never closes and is always open. And the book of your life never ends, and there is always another exciting chapter ahead.

- To be silent at a deep level to hear the most beautiful music coming from colors and things you never thought could make any sound.

- Your dog and cat are some of the smartest beings in your life.

- To see life and the pulsating energy in everything and everyone and to know in the end we are all energy, and there is no end, just energy and new pulsating beginnings.

- We love walking each other home every day.

- To know we are immortal and see and recognize this now!

Wishing you joy on your journey!

Dedication to Maria Sabina

TEACHER OF SACRED MUSHROOM MEDICINE

We would not really have known of Maria Sabina Magdalena Garcia, who was a Mazatec curandera shaman and poet who lived in Huautla de Jimenez, a town in the Sierra Mazateca area of the Mexican state of Oaxaca in southern Mexico, unless, in 1955 a banker and amateur mycologist named R. Gordon Wasson and his wife Valentina (Tina) Pavlovna Guercken-Wasson had visited her. Tina was a pediatrician and although often not credited, Tina worked alongside her husband until her death in 1958. Tina was responsible for introducing her husband to mushrooms. Beginning in 1953, Tina led expeditions with her husband to research the religious use of mushrooms by the native peoples. It was in Mexico where the couple were the first Westerners to witness a psilocybin mushroom ceremony. It was during a later visit, they participated in a velada-healing ceremony led by Maria Sabina.

THE DISCOVERY OF PSILOCYBE MEXICANA

The Wasson's gathered spores from the Psilocybe mexicana that was used in the ceremony and had taken them to Europe where they were cultivated. These mushrooms ended up being examined by Albert Hofmann, resulting in his discovery and isolation of psilocybin and psilocin.

The Wasson's sampled the mushroom ceremony after convincing Maria Sabina they needed her help finding their son, which was unfortunately a false pretense. Maria introduced the Wasson's to her mushroom ceremony. Two years later R. Gordon

Wasson published an article in 1957 *Life* magazine revealing his mushroom journey. The outcome was not good for Maria Sabina as many hundreds traveled to her small village in Oaxaca from around the world to sample her sacred journey on the mushrooms, including Bob Dylan and John Lennon.

MARIA SABINA SUFFERED

The sacred ritual was exposed to the world and Maria Sabina suffered for her innocent revelation. At one point she was put into jail and her house was burned down by the people in her village who were angry at all the people coming and looking for Sabina and the mushrooms. Eventually, her honor was restored. After many years Sabina is now revered and celebrated for her healing mushroom wisdom.

Maria Sabina's life spanned from 1894 to 1985, when she passed away at the age of ninety-one years old. This one tiny woman, with her small brown mushrooms, Psilocybe mexicana, had an enormous impact on the world of brain science. Her invitation into her small sacred mushroom ceremonies lifts our minds today to the potential of healing our mind, body, and soul sickness and the change of our world.

Maria Sabina was a poet and used many "I Am" statements so beautifully in her healing chants during her healing mushroom ceremonies. I had my first exposure to her poems and chants during my MDMA training with MAPS in 2021. I had an assignment to watch her on YouTube and write my response to her way of using plant medicine in healing ceremonies.

During the ceremonies, she sang and recited in a trance-like fashion. She would often say, "I am a woman of light, I am a woman of day" in her Mazatec language. Her healing chants were often spoken during her ceremonies, over the person, while she was performing her healing rituals with the psilocybin mushrooms. I felt so intimately close to Maria Sabina, meeting her through these old films. I found her chanting was a sacred initiation and invitation into the mystical realms.

Because of Maria Sabina's strength of spirit and courage, tenacity, and her willingness to share her healing knowledge of the sacred mushrooms, what she called "her children," we are participating in this work today. I am deeply grateful for her wisdom and spirit and seek to do my best in some humble way to follow her and continue her lineage of healing through psychedelic medicine, rituals, and ceremonies of healing. My spirit has been uplifted and healed in ways I could not begin to imagine because of Maria Sabina and her healing mushroom ceremonies. In her spirit of love and oneness for the healing transformational journey, I dedicate my book to Maria Sabina.

Personal Book Dedication

On my journey through this lifetime, I have been uplifted by many generations of my ancestors who shared their love and wisdom. I still feel their medicine in my bones. They continue to communicate with me through dreams. Their love is eternal and truly continues to inspire me daily.

Friends have been a glorious part of my journey, and many have read these pages and given me valuable feedback. One longtime friend for decades is Laura Kay, who is my Spirit Sister. Her creative and detailed feedback permeates these pages like the gentle fragrance of a rose. She is an excellent sounding board and writing companion. I am deeply grateful for your supportive friendship Laura!

My friend and Soul Sister, Fabiana da Silva Alves, came into my life more recently when we met during the MDMA training we attended through the Multidisciplinary Association of Psychedelic Studies (MAPS) 2021. We had an instant connection that must have spanned far beyond this space and time, and our love and passion for the work with psychedelics is only surpassed by the love we share for one another in our friendship. Fabiana, you are a powerful and insightful woman who enriches my life daily and has inspired my writing, thank you!

I am deeply grateful to the Multidisciplinary Association of Psychedelic Studies (MAPS) for being the catalyst for so much healing in the world, thanks to Rick Doblin and his tenacity and spirit! Rarely can it be said that one person did so much to change so many people, and that is the legacy of Rick Doblin. Thank you, Rick, for changing my life in glorious ways and I get to do the work I love because of you. Of course, you would say it was the whole team, and truly MAPS is a mighty team! So many minds and hearts joined together. Thanks to all the MAPS Team, teachers, facilitators, and leaders!

My longtime editor and friend, Christine Belleris, is the deeply caring and talented Editor and Chief for Health Communication. Christine has worked with me now for thirty years and we produced five books together. She graciously introduced me to my new publisher, Lisa Hagan, and I am now with Lisa Hagan Books. What total bliss for me to work with two brilliant and successful literary women. Thank you, Christine!

Special thanks and appreciation to my son, Joshua Clayton who is a New York-based artist and a professor at NYU in the Department of Computer Science for his encouragement and feedback on the book cover and subtitle. Your love and unwavering support mean the world to me, Josh!

Appreciation to Haley Rivera for the feedback on the Shadow section of the book and the importance of doing the inner healing work with these energies.

I also want to thank Hay House and the Writers Community. Tremendous gratitude to Reid Tracey and Kelly Notaras for their excellent guidance and instruction. I submitted my book proposal for the Hay House contest and came out at the top of the list for "Honorable Mention. As a result, I was noticed by Lisa Hagan Books and then signed with her. Reid and Kelly were highly instrumental in my getting this publishing contract. Thank you, Reid and Kelly, it really works!

My new publisher, Lisa Hagan, is a dynamic woman with a radiant spirit, who has a wonderful way of bringing out the very best in every word, crafting every sentence, and enhancing the look and feel of every page. The energy and love Lisa pours into her work is deeply felt and leaps off the page right into your heart. I am excited and profoundly thankful to be working with her team! What a joy to work with you Lisa and have lots of fun doing our literary craft together. Thank you!

I have an amazing husband, David Grigas, who helps to fill my cup every day with love. After twenty-three years of marriage, it is still getting better every day because we keep growing in love and wisdom daily. David's inspiration, references from volumes of books, editing, suggestions, listening, debating, and constant support have made this book better. Each page is filled with light and healing energy because I sit in this light and healing energy every day within my home and marriage to David. Thank you for your dedication and love to me and our family. Our shared love shines brightly through these words and heals and uplifts all who read these pages. Additionally, I am so happy to be doing this KAP work with you and co-facilitating groups, workshops, and sessions as a married couple. I love you eternally and forever!

A big shout-out of appreciation to my media team at Dillon Media Group in Ocala, Florida. My website design, videos, business cards, and media materials are all done by them. Thank you to Jeff Dillon, Thomas (TJ) Ready, Clinton Grubbs, Kristina Ackerman, Tyler Bell, and Heather Perez who have been tremendous supporters from day one. Their combined creativity helped me to land this publishing contract and made this book a reality. I am forever grateful to each one of you!

Thank you to all my transformational teachers!

I have studied psychology, health and wellness, dreams, transpersonal psychology, social justice, spirituality, and addiction treatment with so many amazing teachers in my lifetime. I give thanks to one of my best personal teachers, John Bradshaw, who was pivotal in my journey to understanding addictions and healing from the inside. Because I started my journey so young, I have been blessed to have spent time personally sharing meals, talking over ideas, interviewing, cooking dinner, hugging, and having one-to-one experiences with so many remarkable people. I have studied with Ram Das, Marianne Williamson, Gerry Jamplosky, Clarissa Pinkola Estes, Marion Woodman, Robert Johnson, Barbara Walker, Lauren Artess, Steven Halpern, O.C. Smith, Les Brown, Barbara Marx-Hubbard, Marilyn Ferguson, Carol Lynn Pearson, Bishop John Shelby Spong, Marcus Borg, Leo Booth, Bishop Desmond Tutu, Rocco Erico, Raymond Moody, Carolyn Myss, Andrew Harvey, Larry Dosey, Angeles Arien, Patricia Sun, Don Miguel Ruiz, Louise Hay, David Williamson, Robert Knapp, Eric Butterworth, Jack Canfield, Mark Victor Hansen, Alan Cohen, Walter Starky, Melba Colgrove, Peter Mc Williams, Matthew Fox, Bernie Siegel, Jeremy Taylor, Rosa Parks, Wally Amos, Stan Krippner, David Feinstein, Clark Moustakas, Thomas Berry, and so many who have touched my life so deeply. What an honor to have been in their field of consciousness to experience their essence. Additionally, spending time with some of the incredible teachers and facilitators at Esalen, Omega, Unity, and Chautauqua. My heart is overflowing!

Made in United States
Orlando, FL
11 January 2024

42377423R00163